"Destined to be a modern American classic, *Surviving Cancer: Something to Celebrate!* chronicles one man's quest for truth and answers, thoughtfully set against the backdrop of an heroic struggle against an insidious melanoma. Man discovers cancer, man battles cancer, man beats cancer!

This is a story that needs telling, a journey with life lessons for us all. Truly, any of us could suffer this crushing diagnosis any day, and how fortunate we are to have such a road map to help navigate the perilous path. A lesser individual might have demeaned the experience by resorting to pathos and self-pity. Happily, Mr. Epstein opts instead for insight and humor, as well as amazing positivity, and we, his rapt audience, are all the richer for it."

—*John R. Kirtley*

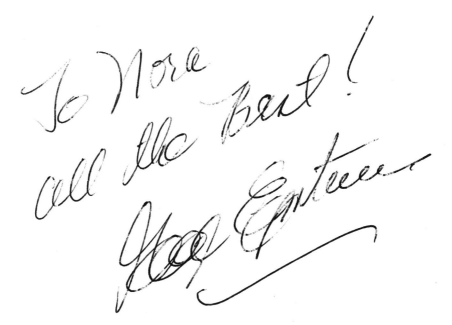

Surviving Cancer
Something to Celebrate!

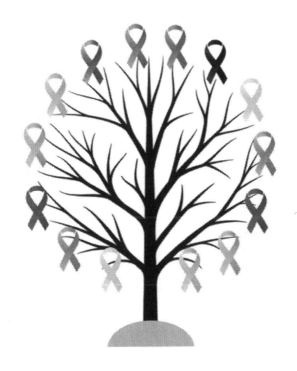

George R. Epstein

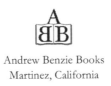

Andrew Benzie Books
Martinez, California

Published by Andrew Benzie Books
www.andrewbenziebooks.com

Printed in the United States of America
First Edition: September 2019

10 9 8 7 6 5 4 3 2 1

Epstien, George R.
Surviving Cancer: Something to Celebrate

ISBN: 978-1-950562-14-5

Cover and book design by Andrew Benzie
www.andrewbenziebooks.com

*This book is dedicated to my wife Janet,
not only for standing by my side through the entire ordeal
of battling melanoma, but for being the rock of my life.*

CONTENTS

PROLOGUE

Twenty-five is the number of kids in a typical elementary school classroom.
It is also the number of players on a major league baseball team's active roster.
It is even the number of one-quarter of our U.S. senators. Most important,
it is the number of people who die every day from melanoma!
—*AIM Melanoma Research*

One cannot help but feel scared and overwhelmed after receiving a melanoma diagnosis. The challenges that patients, caregivers, family members, and friends face can be daunting and can continue even after treatment has ended. I should know as I've been through it all! This is my story.

My early years were spent growing up in the Sunset District of San Francisco. As Mark Twain famously said, "The coldest winter I ever spent was a summer in San Francisco." Well, you can take that to the extreme because the Sunset District almost never saw the sun. It was almost like winter was a year-round season. Not only was it cold most of the time, but if you were waiting to see the sunshine, then it could be a very long time... and at times even depressing. Fortunately, I was just a little kid and didn't know any better. Hey! The gloom from the sky was just about all I ever experienced so it was the norm for me.

In any case, by the time I turned eight years old my family had had enough of the cold weather so we moved from the Sunset District to the East Bay where we finally saw the sun (seemingly for the first time). Hallelujah!

Since seeing the sunshine was a relatively new experience for me, I immediately gravitated to activities where I could spend as much time as possible enjoying the rays beating down on me. After all, I believed that the sun was my new best friend.

Needless to say, growing up in the '50s was an idyllic time for a young kid, never thinking twice about such things as skin cancer— after all, who ever even thought much about it? It was commonplace that I would play in the backyard without a shirt. Harmful rays? What's that? Also, people would bake in the sun at the beach for hours at a time. After all, tan skin was the ultimate picture of health. Or so we thought. People went so far as to go to tanning salons and pay for the privilege of getting "bronzed."

I even remember in comic books when they had a skinny guy who was as white as can be getting sand kicked in his face by some bronze, chiseled guy that looked a lot like Mr. Universe. We thought nothing of being in the sun to enjoy ourselves as much as possible, having no thought of the consequences. The image of this guy was like a picture of health to have a bronze skin (now considered more like leathering). Heck, back in those days it was commonplace for guys to be bare-chested on the beach (and elsewhere), and the girls would even use cocoa butter and reflecting mirrors to get an "attractive" tan as they baked in the sun. Ultimately, we were all in denial that being in the sun wasn't as "sexy" as it was advertised.

Only years later did medical evidence show what a sham it is to be in the sun all the time—but getting cancer from the sun was never a consideration for me growing up back in the 1950s and '60s. I participated in a million outdoor activities, with nary a thought of what the repercussions might be.

Even as a young adult I was in the sun for endless hours, especially during the summer time when I played sports or umpired softball as the sun beat down on me for hours at a time. Even though I wore a shirt and baseball cap, the back of my head was continuously exposed to the sun. Still, I never thought twice about it. Getting skin cancer was never a concern. Using sunscreen was never deemed that necessary. After all, it was the thing to do to be tan and look cool. How stupid. What a dope I was!.

Chapter 1
The Diagnosis

Surviving cancer. It's something to celebrate every day! I'm one of the lucky ones; but it is very likely… perhaps even more than very likely, that for me things could have gone in a completely different direction.

My story begins a number of years ago—the year 2000, to be exact. It was just a day like any other, as I simply went about my usual routine. Then, later that beautiful spring evening I decided to take a shower. It was at this moment that things changed for me, never to be the same. As I washed my hair, I could feel an unusual sensation at the crown of my scalp that simply felt odd. I didn't seem too concerned, because, quite frankly, I was not prepared for what was to come. But my ever-diligent wife Janet decided that this shouldn't be taken lightly and that I should make an appointment with my dermatologist to get it checked out. That's where this tale begins.

It was a glorious day in May, and as Janet and I drove to Kaiser-Pleasanton to visit my dermatologist, Dr. William Liss, I felt no sense of urgency whatsoever. "Just another routine appointment," I thought, and everything would be fine. Now I had visited Dr. Liss back on November 23, 1999, and at that time he detected a minor mole change. It was no big deal; he would make a note of it just to be on the safe side. But that was then. In any case, on this visit, after being called from the waiting room into his office and examined he told me that we should keep an eye on the scalp and then he proceeded to exit the room, leaving me to sit there and twiddle my thumbs. Then, for some reason that remains unclear to me to this day, the doc changed his mind. As he re-entered the room moments later he said, "You know, let's not take any chances. Let's do a biopsy right now."

He then escorted me to an adjoining room where he proceeded to numb my scalp with an anesthetic, and adeptly used his scalpel to operate. Afterwards, he told me to make a follow-up appointment for two weeks down the road, and if anything showed up on the biopsy he would contact me immediately. Okay then, I thought. This sounds like a plan to me. So Janet and I left the office. Janet probably felt a bit uneasy, but I really didn't know what to think so I decided not to speculate, which could only make things worse. So, in hopes of trying to get our minds off whatever prospects might be looming, the two of us went to the local mall for a change of scenery and lunch, which hopefully would be a little uplifting.

Days passed and no word from Dr. Liss. Well, you know what they say… No news is good news, and that certainly applied in this case… or so we thought. Quite frankly, the time flew by as if everything was perfectly fine and dandy. And why wouldn't it be? After all, we would've gotten a call if there were any concerns. Wouldn't we?

Then, on May 26 I was scheduled to see my internist, Dr. Ed Cohen. He's a cool guy, who particularly likes Janet, who always accompanies me on my doctor visits. Dr. Cohen gave me the mandatory routine physical, which, quite bluntly, was the least of my worries. He knew I had seen Dr. Liss and was awaiting the test results, and so gave me advice that, as simple and direct as it was, remains with me to this day: "Hope for the best, but prepare for the worst." Maybe this bit of advice wasn't overly inspiring, but it certainly was realistic.

Two weeks passed, and it was time to revisit Dr. Liss on June 1 for what we thought would be a routine follow-up appointment. No sweat… in… out… on to lunch! So Janet and I were called in to Dr. Liss' office, and we're sitting there patiently waiting… and waiting… and waiting. Usually when the doctor keeps me waiting I get fidgety and start playing with his instruments that are in the room and accessible. No, I don't cough on them or anything like that. Anyway, this time I didn't.

Finally, Dr. Liss comes in the room with a rather stoic look on his face. Uh oh! This can't be good. In any case, he says that he didn't phone us like he said he would because he thought it would be better to tell us the results of the biopsy in person.

"The biopsy shows a central protuberant and ulcerated lesion composed of large spindled and plemorphic melanocytes, extending from the ulcer bed to compress the level III interface, thickness of approximately 5.2 mm," he says. "The ulceration involves approximately 90 percent of the surface. The tumor cells have numerous mitotic figures including atypical forms measuring up to 10 per mm." Huh? In other words, it's a deep metastatic malignant melanoma with high-risk primary. So, to summarize in layman terms: It appears that I'm up shit creek without a paddle.

Each of us sat there for a moment and paused. There was total silence as we tried to absorb all this information. Then Janet somberly asked Dr. Liss, "How long does he have?" I'm not sure I wanted her to ask that question, but now it's out in the open for him to answer. Dr. Liss thought about how to answer her before saying that about seven percent of people with this condition survive as much as a year or so. "Say what? Hey, I didn't even feel bad. That can't be right," I was thinking to myself. Of course I was just thinking this as I didn't actually mutter a word. I guess I was too stunned to say anything, and the last thing I needed to do was contradict the doctor by telling him I think he might be full of crappola. At least I was hoping he was.

Meanwhile, Janet appeared to be in shock as she had lost all the color in her face, so the doc asked her if she wanted to lie down on the examining table, and she meekly nodded in the affirmative.

Dr. Liss then turned off the lights in the room for a few moments in an effort to help Janet regain her composure. During this brief time of silence my mind wandered (as it usually does anyway). I was thinking to myself of an old joke I once heard. In it the doctor says: "The tests show that your cancer is advanced. You have just a few months to live." The patient replies: "But doc, I can't pay off my medical bills in a just few months." So the doctor pauses, and then says: "In that case, I'm giving you an additional six months."

In any case, after several moments of complete silence he then tells Janet and me that he's taken the liberty to schedule an appointment for me on June 5 to see Dr. Barry Rasgon, the head and neck surgeon at Kaiser-Oakland.

Well, there wasn't much else to say. I really didn't have much of a reaction to hearing all of this. I guess I was just a bit numb after learning how totally screwed I was. I think Janet was even more stunned. So what does one do when you get a bit of life-changing devastating news like this? Naturally, we headed to the mall to return a pair of shoes or some such thing, and then went home. Isn't that what anyone would do? There wasn't a great deal of conversation about what we just learned at the doctor's office. Frankly, I didn't believe either one of us truly comprehended the ramifications of what we had just been told. In other words, we were shell-shocked and in a bit of a daze.

What is true is that melanoma, the most dangerous form of skin cancer, is much deadlier when it appears on the scalp or neck than somewhere else on the body. Part of the reason for this is that diagnosis may be delayed because it can be obscured by hair on the scalp, which was what happened in my case. People with scalp or neck melanoma die at nearly twice the rate of those with melanoma elsewhere on the body, the researchers at the University of North Carolina at Chapel Hill found. Conversely, people with melanoma on the arms, legs, face or ears are found to have the best prognosis.

As I lay in bed that night I gazed at the walls and thought, 'Wow, my dad died of melanoma at the age of 76; his mother died of melanoma at the age of 76. And here I am, in my early 60s with this same disease.' I thought for sure I'd make it to at least 76 since I didn't have any of my dad's bad habits… I don't smoke or drink, etc. Heck, I take reasonably good care of myself and I'm not even that big of a jerk! So why is the Big Guy upstairs picking on me? While I'm having this conversation with myself I'm still thinking that this just can't be my time to check out. It just can't be. Hey, maybe I *will* have a drink. Nah!

The next several days Janet and I simply continued to go through the motions of doing our typical daily activities, just waiting until that next appointment. I really didn't know what to expect since all this information regarding the severity of my condition really hadn't sunk in. After all, I felt pretty good; still felt like running around and enjoying life like I always did. But, at the same time, things were now a bit different. Maybe "enjoying life" had taken a different definition for me. I had become more acutely aware of everyday things that up to this point were always considered 'second nature.' In other words, I had stopped taking things—even the smallest of things—for granted. For example, I would actually stop to listen to birds sing, or consciously feel a cool breeze, or any number of other little things that under different circumstances can, and usually are, easily taken for granted. Perhaps, even in a literal sense, I began to "smell the flowers."

When I wasn't around to listen, Janet would call her friends to tell them the early prognosis. One of them, Susie Goldsmith, was gracious enough to volunteer to go with us to my next doctor's appointment to take notes so we could just listen to what would be said without having to worry about absorbing everything at that moment. That was very nice of her and at the time, I thought, not necessary but still awfully gracious. Suzy was very adamant about accompanying us so, hey, when you get an offer like that you just can't turn it down.

So the three of us, Janet, Susie, and I all arrived at Dr. Rasgon's office at Kaiser Oakland on June 5 for my 11:15 a.m. appointment. Having never experienced a medical issue this serious before I really didn't know what to expect the doc to tell me... but I was soon to find out.

Dr. Rasgon entered the room where the three of us were all patiently waiting, and he introduced himself. "This guy's a lot younger than I thought," I said to myself. "Does he really know what he's doing?" Without a lot of explanation, he told me that he's already scheduled surgery for the following day and I should get there early in preparation for them to slice and dice. Whoa, Nellie! Hey, I just met this guy a few minutes ago and already he's setting out to cut my head apart? I don't think so! Meanwhile, Susie was diligently taking notes, and Janet sat there, becoming ever so skeptical. I was also sitting there thinking to myself, 'What's going on here?' So Janet and Susie

Each decided to speak up and told Dr. Rasgon that a second opinion might be in order. 'Here! Here!' I was thinking, and maybe even a third or fourth opinion might be in order while we're at it. So Dr. Rasgon pulls back a bit, and told us of some of the preliminary steps we might take, but at the same time reminding us that time was of the essence. Message received! So everyone took a collective deep breath and we came up with a slightly different game plan. Instead of rushing into a quick surgery, an MRI was ordered and scheduled for June 7, which might reveal a little more detail and information.

So now that the operation has been postponed a bit, it gave us time... albeit very little time... to scramble in an effort to gather more information to enlighten us as much as possible about this disease, its ramifications, and possible treatment options. With no time to waste Janet was able to schedule an appointment at USCF for me to see Dr. Richard W. Sagebiel, who is renowned in the world of pathology, and might be able to shed more light on this subject, of which we knew very little.

The following day, June 6, I got a quick response from the UCSF Clinical Cancer Center welcoming me and confirming my appointment for June 12. I was reminded that the Melanoma Center is set up to address of the needs of newly-diagnosed patients and that, from a medical standpoint, there are many specialties that are important in the evaluation of melanoma. These include Melanoma Pathology, Dermatology, Internal Medicine, Medical Oncology, Surgical Oncology, ENT Surgery and Radiation Therapy.

Clinicians from each of these areas of expertise comprise this multidisciplinary team, and I was told that it is their task to put their heads together to assess my needs and propose a plan of attack that would be tailored specifically for my situation. Wow! I was impressed by the professionalism and depth of scope with which they planned to undertake my diagnosis.

And that wasn't all. They stated that in addition to their focus on the medical aspects of melanoma, they were just as concerned with the emotional impact, the effects it may have on my day-to-day life, and even how it might affect other family members, including how they might adjust to all of this. Part of the visit, I was told, would also include a meeting with the clinical psychologist to discuss whatever concerns or reactions I might be experiencing.

In other words, this program is designed to provide a comprehensive consultation concerning the medical as well as the emotional aspects of having melanoma. Well, I was sold. Their confidence was ever so contagious.

Dr. Liss had written UCSF Dermatology a letter to brief them on my condition. It read: "Mr. Epstein was seen on May 18, 2000 for a nodule on the top of his scalp which had been palpable for about 2 months. He was not certain if something may have been present before that. There was some crusting/bleeding when manipulated. Exam revealed a 1 cm crusted skin colored nodule on the top of the scalp. An excisional biopsy was done at that visit, and the pathology revealed a 5.3mm melanoma, level III. Full body exam was unremarkable. The patient feels well and has no sign of spread. Chest X-ray and screening labs were normal. His family history is significant for his father and grandmother both died of melanoma in their mid-70s."

CHAPTER 2
DOING THE RESEARCH

However, in the meantime, before I would go to UCSF, I scrambled to do a little research of my own, and was able to gather the names and phone numbers of some of the leading melanoma research experts in the world, including such oncology gurus as Dr. John Kirkwood at the University of Pittsburgh Cancer Center (an adjuvant of high-dose interferon which he feels is significant in increasing survival in advanced melanoma); Dr. Kim Margolin, a melanoma expert at City of Hope in Duarte, California; Dr. John Glaspy at UCLA's Jonsson Comprehensive Cancer Center; Dr. Jeff Webber at the Kenneth Norris Jr. Cancer Center at USC; Dr. Donald Morton at the John Wayne Cancer institute in Los Angeles; Lynn Spitler at St. Francis Hospital in San Francisco, as well as experts at Sloan-Kettering Cancer Center in New York; M.D. Anderson Cancer Center in Houston, Texas; Mayo Clinic Cancer Center in Minnesota; etc. I intended to get in touch with each of them… well, okay, realistically, maybe just some of them, and pick their brains in order to find out what the latest treatments were in fighting this disease.

Within a couple of days, after a slew of phone calls, more phone calls, and then even more phone calls, I actually became quite a bit more knowledgeable, as I learned from many of the experts that there is no magic bullet in fighting this disease. Furthermore, the case studies which had already been conducted had, by and large, all proven to give marginal results. Still, there were a myriad of clinical trials and a couple of stand-by methods whose results seemed to be just slightly more predictable than a blind crapshoot.

11

In any case, this research proved to be a very time-consuming project, but I figured that's a good thing. Strange as it sounds, the phone research process actually helped to take my mind off myself. What I found out is that there were so many choices. The truth is that today, after many years of the "same old, same old" treatments which produced questionable value, there have finally been significant and meaningful advances in melanoma research, including promising results with new drugs and combinations in clinical trials. Quite frankly, it's all very confusing, especially since even the 'experts' don't really know or agree on what works and what doesn't. I guess that's why they call them "clinical trials"—so patients who are so vulnerable act as guinea pigs.

The alternative to these choices was the standard protocol, which is a program of injections of Melicine and Interferon. There were two different ways to go here, as proposed by UC Irvine. The first involved two injections a week for four weeks; and then two injections every two months thereafter for two years. The other option was for a higher dose of Interferon every day for four weeks; then a lower dose taken three times a week thereafter for the next 11 months. Or I could roll the dice and get enrolled in one of the many clinical trials as some of the doctors had been recommending. *Hmmmmm…* tough choice.

According to the National Cancer Institute's (NCI) cancer information database, some, but not all, clinical trials are supported by hospitals, medical centers, or even drug companies. Each trial enrolls people with certain specific characteristics, which are called "entry criteria" or "eligibility criteria." A patient's doctor can determine whether the patient meets the eligibility requirements and whether taking part in a trial is an appropriate option. The National Institute of Health

has published a pamphlet entitled "Taking Part in Clinical Trials— What Cancer Patients Need to Know." I highly recommend that one reads it before deciding to participate in one of these trials as it is very enlightening. Part of me felt like a "guinea pig" in these clinical trials being used to test less-than-reliable options, and merely hoping for a positive outcome. Talk about the ultimate crapshoot with so much at stake!

Actually, it's the first step in developing a game plan, and deciding what are the most appropriate recommendations once a diagnosis is reached. Questions that need to be asked include: What are the current best treatment options, and why do/don't you use or recommend interferon like UCSF? Are the recommended treatments more aggressive, and what kind of improvement can be expected? What are the cutting edge treatments? What are the side effects of these treatments? And what clinical trials might I be a candidate for? I found that the answers to each of these questions varied considerably from place to place.

In any case, June 7 arrived and I went in for my MRI, hoping beyond hope that all their previous findings were just a big mistake, and that everything was going to be fine—yeah, right! In my heart I knew better, but I guessed it didn't hurt to dream just a little. After all, maybe… just maybe I might have been part of that seven percent who survive this ordeal.

In any case, I knew I wasn't kidding myself. So, it's back to reality. If you've never had an MRI before then the first time can be a rude awakening, especially if you're at all claustrophobic. Without going into detail, you disrobe and they lay you on this table and slide you into this long, narrow tube. It reminds me of that scene in the movie "The Great Escape" when Charles Bronson was digging a tunnel to escape from the prisoner-of-war camp in Nazi Germany, and he felt like the world was closing in on him. Well, it's something like that, except without the Nazis. In any case, about 45 minutes later it was all over and I just had to await the results, which would be sent to Dr. Rasgon.

As it happened, the results came sooner than later, and Dr. Rasgon called to let me know that they were inconclusive. So he took the liberty to schedule another test, a C.T. Scan on June 9, which might serve us better by revealing more.

Things were moving pretty quickly at this point. They had to, and because of the pace things were going there was no time for any emotions to get in the way, which was just as well.

So the following day, June 8, I was scheduled to go to the Pre-Surgery Center where Dr. Rasgon was to perform a reexcision and sentinel lymph node biopsy. It was preceded by a pre-op lymphscintigram, where radioactive dye was injected in the nuclear medicine department. I was awake for this part of the procedure. It really wasn't a big deal, or at least it didn't seem that way to me. As I'm on the table ready for this procedure, Dr. Rasgon decided this would make a great teaching moment, and took great pleasure in describing what he was doing, blow-by-blow, to Janet, who was nearby. I was lying on this table while Dr. Rasgon was performing his duties.

Janet sat next to him, and the two of them seemed to be having quite the time. He was explaining what he was doing while Janet seemed to be thoroughly intrigued. I sure liked being the subject of what seems like a science experiment… *not!*

Again, while I'm all for increasing one's knowledge, was this really the time and place? I guess so.

Then, I was wheeled in for the biopsy where a blue dye was injected to isolate the sentinel nodes. Wide local excisions under general anesthesia were performed to make certain that the margins were covered. Dr. Rasgon looked under the gamma camera and it was revealed that there was one "hot" lymph node.

The results wouldn't be known for a few days, as I was then wheeled to the recovery room.

My head was bandaged so that I looked like a fortune-telling gypsy swami, except that I didn't have a crystal ball to gaze into to predict anyone's future, let alone my own.

Still, I was released from the hospital with this very chic and stylist headgear resembling a turban, which I'm certain was quite attractive. Perhaps it might catch on as the latest fashion statement, but I rather doubted it. I was to get a lot of rest, and not exert myself. I took that to mean no helping around the house doing stuff like, well you know… picking up clothes, putting things away, doing dishes… in other words, things that require a little bit of exertion. It's not something I'm that fond of doing anyway so, hey, at least there was that perk.

Dr. Rasgon concluded that there was no point messing around with a "hot" lymph node that could eventually spread throughout my system, so a subsequent surgery would be needed... and pronto. It was quickly settled that July 6 would be the date to take action.

However, before the July 6 date of my surgery there was a very important event—my son Evan's high school graduation ceremony. I've been told to rest, but there was no way I was going to miss this event.

Still on the agenda, I went in for a CT Scan at the Radiology Department. The results of this follow-up CT scan of the neck, chest, abdomen and pelvis showed a 1 cm subcutaneous nodule in the left retroauricular area. The remainder of the scan was negative. This was to be my last official Kaiser visit for awhile so I could focus, if you could call it that, on Evan's impending big day.

My son's high school graduation day finally came, and the ceremony was held in a nearby public park with lawn seating very limited. Janet left home early to get a good spot, and it was arranged for my friend Susie Goldsmith to pick me up, as her son and mine are best friends and were both part of the graduating class. So I dragged myself out of bed, got dressed and headed out the door. I then ever-so-slowly got myself from the car to the park, as I was pretty wiped out from a lack of energy (something I knew I had better get used to). We all met up with Janet as she had found a nice lawn spot where they had spread a blanket to witness the proceedings. Wearing this turban-like headdress made me mildly self-conscious (I looked ridiculous, really), since I was sure that I was drawing some stares. But then I thought, 'Hey, I really don't know these people, so why should I care that I look goofy? They're not here to see me, and vice versa.'

During the ceremony I sat on the park lawn and watched the procession of graduates being introduced and called up to the podium to receive their diplomas. It was really quite a moment to know that your kid is now ready to move on to the next stage of his life—and won't be around for you to nag any longer... and vice versa. Touching, indeed.

Before I knew it, this festive day of jubilation ends, Evan was now officially a high school graduate, and reality began to set in. The very next day I was back at Kaiser Oakland for a post-op session where I met with Dr. Hilsinger, the chief of Kaiser's Head and Neck Department, to get sutures removed from the biopsy.

From that day on to my surgery date I had to lay low (literally, most of the time) and tried not to get too nervous or panicky. I knew that if I showed signs of nervousness then it would just make things harder for Janet, whom I'm sure was already nervous enough for the both of us.

It was clear that I was not out of the woods so when I next met with Dr. Rasgon, it was to discuss the results of the biopsy and to make sure we were both on the same page. He advised me to get a full-body PET scan, which would undoubtedly serve my cause better in determining whether or not the melanoma had spread. This was another instance of Dr. Rasgon wanting to leave no stone unturned (he's a perfectionist if ever there was one—that's a good thing!). Interestingly, Kaiser Hospital didn't at that time have the capacity to offer PET scans so Dr. Rasgon used his influence by making arrangements for me to go to the VA Hospital in Palo Alto. There was no eating that day, and I was to bring a brief medical history.

As luck would have it, one of Janet's old college friends, Barbara Friedenthal, and her husband Ron, live in the Palo Alto area, so Janet called her to tell her the scoop. Barbara, always the kind soul and good friend, offered to have us stay over the night of the test since we would undoubtedly be too exhausted to return home that same day. It turned out to be a good move.

Days later we headed to the VA Hospital, allowing time to sign all the preparatory paperwork that was involved. I found it ironic that upon my arrival the first question that was asked by some straight-laced receptionist was: "Did the doctor order this test?" That's a real gem. Now I understand that the person asking this question was just doing her job. I know she didn't make up this question and so it's undoubtedly not her fault that she had to ask it. So, I paused for what seemed like an infinite amount of time as I carefully considered how to properly answer this question in regard to a PET scan. After all, this is a full body scan that helps them detect where the cancer is in your body and is part of the process of staging the cancer. Well, what I could have answered was: "No, the doctor didn't order this test. I just want to waste two and a half hours of my day, spend the prior twenty-four hours with no eating allowed whatsoever because I have nothing better to do with my time. And I love drinking the barium 'smoothies' and being injected with radioactive dye because I'm hoping to develop some other type of cancer years from now from all of the radiation exposure. I live close to a power plant but I don't think I'm getting my daily intake of radiation exposure. While I'm at it, I didn't get prior authorization from my insurance company because I want to shell out thousands of dollars out of pocket for this test because I'm not in enough credit card debt and am hoping to claim bankruptcy before the end of the year." Really? Was she kidding? At least that's what I should have said.

In any case, after a bit of a wait (which always makes one's mind go in a thousand different directions) they wheeled me to the area where they conducted the scan. I stripped and they laid me on a table. Geez, I'm lying on this table and, just as I recalled from the recent past, I felt just like I was some sort of medical experiment. In any case, they gave me this injection and told me to lie still for what seemed like an eternity. Then I'm rolled into the scanning room on a gurney. In the midst of the scan, all of a sudden I had to go to the bathroom like nobody's business. Just then the technician reminded me to be still. Good timing! Somehow, I got through the scan without much of a ruckus, and no damage done, test-wise or personally. Whew!

It's amazing how quickly the test results can be obtained.

They were almost immediate. As it turned out the results showed an "increased uptake in the left retroauricular area, measuring 1.3 cm in size. It also found a right iliac lymph node uptake, measuring 1.0 cm." The results were then forwarded to Dr. Rasgon for analysis. He was then to determine the next step to take.

In the meantime, I got dressed and Janet and I, now pretty exhausted, headed on over to Barbara F's, where she had everything ready for our arrival. I headed right to her couch in front of the TV and almost immediately fell asleep (something I'd probably do at her house under almost any other circumstances, but that's okay because she knew I was able to completely relax there). Man, was I out of it. The rest of the day was a total blank. I was completely zonked. Let's face it; I know that I can be a real couch potato without much prodding. But seriously, I didn't remember getting off that couch, eating anything, doing anything... absolutely nada! Homer Simpson has nothing on me.

The following morning Janet and I headed home. I'm sure Barbara and Ron thought I was a fantastic guest. Basically, all I did was sleep on their couch. One might say that I was the 'perfect guest.' After all, I didn't have any complaints or constant demands. On the other hand, it could be argued that I probably wasn't the most stimulating conversationalist, but, hey—my behavior wasn't much different than other times that I've been to their house when I've dosed off on their couch (to this day it's the most comfortable one on which I've ever had the pleasure of plotzing).

Just a few days passed and next on the agenda was a consultation visit at the UCSF/Mt. Zion Melanoma Center in San Francisco with the Multidisciplinary Panel, headed by co-directors Richard Sagebiel and Mohammed Kashani-Sabet. Its purpose was to get a second opinion in terms of further treatment for my condition. What's notable is that my father died of melanoma in 1992 at the age of 76; and his mother was also diagnosed with skin cancer.

Now here's the part I liked: Upon review, they concluded that (in their words): "he is a well appearing gentleman..." I didn't absorb the remainder of what they said; I was too dazzled by their seemingly accurate assessment... if I humbly do say so myself.

Actually, they spent time reviewing the biopsy from May 18 and interpreted the result as a malignant melanoma, 5.0mm in thickness, Clark level III, with 90 percent of the tumor ulcerated, moderate angiogenesis present, high mitotic rate of ten mitoses per high powered field.

After deciphering all the rest of the mumbo-jumbo, the bottom line was this: "Based on the UCSF/Mt. Zion Melanoma Center database, this is considered a high-risk primary lesion, with a five-year overall survival of less than 50 percent." Wow, that sounded a little depressing. Or at least it should to a normal soul. On the other hand, it was better than just seven percent survival probability for one year. In any case, my reaction was surprisingly not being depressed. Instead, it was more like: "Oh yeah… we'll see about that!"

It reminded me of the joke when three buddies were talking about death and dying. One asked: "When you're in your casket and friends and family are mourning you, what would you like to hear them say about you?" The first guy says," I would like to hear them say that I was a great family man." The second man then says," I would like to hear that I was a wonderful husband and philanthropist who made a difference in our children of tomorrow." The last guy then says, "I would like to hear them say: 'Look, he's moving!'"

A few days later it was back to the business of attempting to get to the bottom of things as we headed over to UCSF once again. What an interesting, if not bizarre visit it turned out to be. First Dr. Mohammed Kashani-Sabet, a renowned expert in the field of dermatology and Co-Director of UCSF's Melanoma Center, introduced himself, and then told me that a series of other doctors would be taking a look at me, one by one. Really?

So had it come down to me being the center of a medical freak show that all these people are going to take turns gawking at? Apparently so.

That's right—the circus was in town! Come one, come all—come see the freak and take your turn staring, poking and prodding to your heart's content! All that was missing was a ringmaster to announce each of the medical experts as they entered the room in single file to take their turn checking out the medical dummy in the room. They must have had so much fun!

Well, after all the tests and probing was finished, the experts huddled together, and the long and short of it came down to this: I had a "central protuberant and ulcerated lesion composed of large spindled and pleomorphic melanocytes, extending from the ulcer bed to compress the level III interface, thickness of approximately 5.2 mm. The ulceration involved approximately 90 percent of the surface. The tumor cells had numerous mitotic figures including atypical forms measuring up to 10 per mm."

The final diagnosis by Dr. Richard Sagebiel, Clinical Professor of Pathology and Dermatology at UCSF, was as follows: Malignant melanoma, nodular protuberant type, invasive to 5.0 mm (level III) with ulceration, high mitotic rate, high risk primary. Well, I knew that the seriousness of everything was more than my just having an infected pimple, but nonetheless, this result did *not* sound good at all! It was time to take a deep breath and let it all sink in.

CHAPTER 3
SEEING THE SHRINK

A few days passed, but before I was to have this major surgery I was told I must meet with a Kaiser psychologist to address my emotional well-being or some such nonsense. I guessed they were concerned about any trepidations I may have had about the impending procedure and my future outlook, whatever that may have been. So, I was told to schedule an appointment to go to Kaiser's mental ward or what I fondly called the "looney bin" or the "nuthouse." No disrespect to those who may be truly crazy, but when I was there all I could think about was the film "One Flew Over The Cuckoo's Nest." But I diverge. Anyway, it is there that I met with one of the Kaiser psychologists to see if I was stable... or maybe I should be committed? I really had absolutely no idea why I was here, but while I'm kept waiting in this shrink's office, staring at the couch, I perused the room, reading all this guy's academic certificates posted on the walls.

Finally he walked in—an older gentleman with a beard. "Oh, it's Kris Kringle," I surmised since he reminded me of actor Edmund Gwenn from the film classic "Miracle on 34th Street." In any case, he introduced himself to me, but before he could ask me any questions about myself, I began to ask him about himself. 'So, you graduated from Podunk U.? What made you go into psychology? Did you have personal problems that needed to be addressed?' I just kept at it nonstop with a barrage of questions about himself, his background, and what he found most satisfying about being a psychologist.

I believe that all the questions directed his way threw him for a bit of a loop, catching him off-balance. After all, we were on his turf and he's the one supposed to be asking the questions. In any case, before he had a chance to ask much about me, the patient, he looked at his watch and said," Well, that's all we've got time for today." And that was the end of what was obviously a very meaningful and satisfying session!

So much for getting to my inner being and retrieving all the pent-up feelings I might be experiencing. Perhaps I got this guy thinking to himself, asking exactly why he decided to go into psychology. It certainly wasn't to put up with guys like me.

Quite frankly, I've always wondered what makes people go into the field of psychology. For example, do they think they can discover the root of their own issues by talking to enough mental patients? I'm guessing that having a patient like me might have one second-guessing one's decision to become a psychologist in the first place. And for good reason!

In any case, four days later I met with Dr. Rasgon once again, this time to review the results of the biopsy. There was one positive node, so, not to take any chances, it became a foregone conclusion: surgery was a must if I was to have any chance at survival. And there was little time to waste. So the surgery was scheduled right then and there, and it was time to roll the dice.

A surgery date was finally set. Well, so much for having a leisurely, festive, fun-filled 4th of July. For the days, and especially nights, leading up to "the big day" I spent considerable time in bed just gazing up at the ceiling, and quite frankly, reminding myself of my grandmother's approach to potentially traumatic experiences and such things. She was a fatalist, and I guess I am too. Instead of thinking "why me?" I just approached it in the same vein as my internist, Dr. Ed Cohen, who told me: "Hope for the best, but prepare for the worst." That's sage advice, indeed. I knew there was not much I could really do about my fate at this point since it was pretty much in the hands of Dr. Rasgon (not that there was any pressure on him, mind you). So, strange as it seemed, I remained pretty calm.

Time marched on as I had an appointment to see Dr. Cohen and also scheduled a follow-up session with Dr. Rasgon, who recommended that I set up an appointment with one of the oncologists to discuss post-surgery treatment options. He told me a little bit about each of the doctors in that department and he suggested I see Dr. James Simons, as he felt our two personalities offered a good chance of us meshing as a team. So let's be honest, it takes real teamwork to come up with a solution to fight the after-affects of melanoma.

Dr. Rasgon also mentioned that Kaiser offered a support group for cancer patients so that they may talk about their specific conditions and have the opportunity to air their concerns. Janet thought it might be a good idea for me to check it out. I wasn't convinced. But Janet won out (as usual), so I decided to go.

The next day, one day before I went in for a preliminary checkup at the pre-surgery center, I attended one of the Cancer Supportive Care Classes at Kaiser, which included a topic of the day plus a question and answer session with a Kaiser Permanente oncologist. It was more of a generic class, and as it turned out, I was the only melanoma patient present. Still, the topics varied each session, and included such things as "Treatment Decisions & Second Opinions;" "What's New and Interesting: An Update from the American Society of Clinical Oncologists;" "Biofeedback: Practical Ways to Lower Stress and Pain;" "Mind, Body & Spirit: Approaches to Wellness;" "The Fighting Spirit: Engaging Your Inner Fire;" etc. There was some good stuff offered here. It was just a matter of picking and choosing what pertains to your personal circumstances. For many, these sessions are a blessing. It serves as an opportunity for some to vent and express their concerns. It's especially important for those who have no built-in support system, such as family or close friends with whom they can share the stress they are going through. Fortunately, I didn't fit into that category since I could unload all my crap onto Janet whenever I wanted.

Time marched on, and before you knew it, it was the day before the big Fourth of July weekend and I had scheduled an appointment to consult with Dr. James Simons to find out if he had some magic pill I could take to make this all go away. Hey, I was just thinking out loud. One can always hope, no matter how ridiculous it may be. In any case, Dr. Simons and I hit it off almost immediately. I think the fact that Janet came with me helped turn the tide. He might have been listening to what I had to say, but he was looking at Janet the entire time (I couldn't blame him). You can draw whatever conclusions you want from that. I guess I was looking for a bookie's insight that might tell me what treatment gave me better odds in dealing with melanoma. Still, while Dr. Simons admitted that he couldn't do that, he was at least honest in saying that he really was uncertain if any treatment might be better than any other I might choose. In other words, it was just a matter of rolling the dice, and it was strictly my call. I'd have to give it some serious thought. It was food for thought that I better take seriously because I had to deal with it for the duration. But at this specific moment in time I believe I needed a diversion as all of this was piling up and becoming exhausting. For this, the timing couldn't have been better.

The Fourth of July has always been one of my favorite holidays— the pageantry, the barbecue, the fireworks, and best of all, the company. It's great having everyone for a get-together and this year, in particular, it was an opportunity to get my mind off my troubles and impending procedure, and all that was to follow. I guess it's times like these that just make one appreciate what life is all about. Unfortunately, the holiday was just too short. I find that holidays are like the movies—the really good ones are never long enough.

CHAPTER 4
D-DAY ARRIVES

The Fourth of July holiday came and went almost quicker than the blink of an eye, so now it was back to reality as "The Day" finally arrived. It was time for surgery. I was given pre-op instructions and arrived at Kaiser Oakland sometime near dawn to await further instructions. While in the changing room, there came a knock on the door; it was none other than Bill Fleck, one of Janet's friends who, among other things, drives the bus for her senior excursions (Janet runs the Seniors Program for the City of Piedmont Recreation Department). Bill also happens to be a chaplain, and he arrived to show support and to say a few prayers for me. Geez, I hoped it was not my last rites! Then they carted me away to the operating room where the anesthesiologist did his thing and told me to count from one hundred backwards. I believe that by the time I got to 98 I was out like a light.

In the meantime, Janet was in the waiting room, sitting nervously with all her thoughts. Knowing Janet as I do, it was clear that this was not an easy time for her. Luckily, she had company; a few friends who tried to keep her as upbeat as possible. After all, it's times like these that show who your real friends are.

While Janet was nervously sitting in the waiting room and I was in the operating room, there came a booming voice over the hospital's loudspeaker calling out Janet's name. Well, to understand my wife you need to know that she often thinks of the glass as "half-empty"—in other words, thinking the worst. Anyway, she was jolted when they called her name, and immediately feared what could come next—that the doctor was reporting that I had croaked right there on the operating table! Still, Janet gathered her strength just enough to get up from her chair and went right to the waiting room desk, only to be told that she had a telephone call from my sister, Darlene. Darlene was simply "checking in " to see how everything was going. I can't tell you how relieved Janet was that it was really nothing more than a benign phone call asking about my status. Still, it scared the hell out of her. Hey, what I can't figure out is how someone could even get the telephone number of the waiting room to have someone paged?

During this period I'm in la-la land, completely out of it. Obviously the anesthesiologist did a great job, as during the entire 2-1/2 hour surgery I was gone like three sheets to the wind.

It was only after the fact that I learned of the complete description of the procedure. It went something like this: The patient (that would be me) was taken to the operating room and monitored for general anesthesia. General endotracheal anesthesia was induced. The patient was the placed in the prone position with appropriate padding. The previous melanoma was injected in Nuclear Medicine and scanned with technetium-99. This localized two sentinel lymph nodes in the posterior occipital areas and PET scan previously localized a left posterior mastoid area node.

Attention was first turned toward this node and a skin incision was made with a 15 blade and an en bloc dissection of all the likely fibrofatty tissue was undertaken with Bovie cautery and periosteal elevators. This was then examined on the back table and the lymph nodes in question were found.

Attention was then turned toward the sentinel node.

Lymphazurin dye was injected around the previous melanoma incision. Approximately 0.5 cc was used and posterior occipital incisions were made, looking for the sentinel lymph nodes. The gamma-probe was then used to help localize the nodes and hot spots. An en bloc resection approach was taken and the fibrofatty lymph node-bearing tissue was resected and on the back table the sentinel lymph nodes were localized with the gamma-probe. This was done bilaterally.

In layman's terms, during the posterior lateral neck excision a grand total of 52 lymph nodes were removed from my neck region. Fifty-two lymph nodes! Now that's a lot of nodes, no matter how you slice it! Dr. Rasgon made it perfectly clear that he wasn't going to take any chances that the melanoma might spread. He was determined to nip it in the bud. Way to go, doc! I'm with you all the way on this one.

A 2 cm margin was taken around it and the wound was then closed with .1-0 Maxon and staples. The other three incisions were closed with 4-0 chromic and staples as well. Bacitracin was placed on the wound. After all was said and done, I was returned to the recovery room in good condition, or so they say.

The next period of time was a little foggy (I wonder why?). Best as I can remember, I awoke in the recovery room rather slowly. After that it still seems like a blur.

Later, I'm wheeled up to my hospital room, where I spend the night to recoup. I was all bandaged up and, quite frankly, I looked like a mummy, with bandages all over my head, neck and shoulder. Everything was all still numb, but I was feeling no pain. Then the nurse came in and attached an IV to the back of my hand. Wow! All of a sudden I went from a semi-stupor state to one of intense pain. Son of a b…. *errr*, gun! Well, then the nurse's aide left the room so I'm stuck there… literally. This needle stuck in the back of my hand was causing my hand to throb like hell. What a fine how-do-you-do this was!

You know, it sure seems ironic. I go through this entire invasive procedure (admittedly in a state of unconsciousness) in which they slice me open and tear out all those nodes, and I get through it pretty well. Then something that seems so trivial as injecting an IV causes such great pain. It just doesn't seem right.

Luckily, later that evening I was treated to a surprise visit. Dr. Rasgon came to my room to see how I was doing. That was unexpected, and quite frankly, I thought, pretty cool. This guy's had a long day slicing and dicing in the surgery room, and yet found the time to check in on me. He told me he was taking a break and thought he'd see how I'm doing. So he sat down, and we started chewing the fat about anything and everything. It was all good. Then

I told him how much this IV was bothering me and in the bat of an eye he paged the nurse's aide and told her to remove it from my hand. What a relief! Before leaving, he told me to get some rest, and let me know that I was to be released to go home the next morning.

Well, getting *real* rest was easier said than done. Apparently my room was right near the floor's nursing station, which seemed to become the gathering place for gabbing sessions. And, with my door open, these gab fests took place throughout the night. Still, it was only one night, and, frankly, under the circumstances of what might have been, I felt pretty fortunate. Hey, loud yakking or no loud yakking by the staff, it was all good.

Somehow, I got through the night, and the next day I was scheduled for release. As Dr. Martin Luther King aptly put it, "Free at last, free at last, thank God Almighty, I'm free at last!"… or something like that. At least that's the way I felt about going home.

After dressing and getting my release papers, it was time to head home. At this point I was still trying to process all that just took place in the past 24 hours and figure out what effects it was going to have on me.

Upon arriving home there awaited an unexpected gift for me at the back door. It was a welcome home token from Aileen Frankel, someone, to this point, I really didn't know that well, but was herself a melanoma survivor. Well, how thoughtful of her. As it turned out, this gracious gesture became the beginning of what has turned out to be a wonderful and long-lasting friendship that continues to this day.

A gesture like this can't be ignored so I gave Aileen a phone call to thank her for her thoughtfulness. We got to chatting, and she gave me an abbreviated synopsis of her ordeal with melanoma and let me know about a UCSF cancer support group whose sessions she was attending. She asked if I was interested in checking it out. Knowing I had nothing to lose

I thought "why not?" Aileen told me that she would get all the details and let me know when and where the next meeting was to take place.

Time marched on as it had been just a week since the operation, and I was back to see Dr. Rasgon for a post-op "look-see." He took one look at me, as if I was the latest version of Mr. Potato Head, and could see that things weren't just right. So he decided to set me up for physical therapy treatment because it looked like my head wasn't screwed on straight. No, seriously, my head was literally tilted to one side as I seemed to, unwittingly, lean to the left. I didn't even realize that I was doing it. It was no big deal, but I didn't want to go around looking like a marionette doll that needed its strings pulled to have my head on straight. So I agreed that, as my father-in-law would say, "it couldn't hoit!"

A bit later, I went to see Dr. D.D. Cheung for suture removal. It was quick and painless and I was beginning to feel a little bit like my old self again. Yes, a mark was left from the crown of my scalp to the base of my neck, but that was the least of my worries. I wasn't going to win any beauty pageant awards anyway so what was the big deal?

Later that same evening Susie Goldsmith, who had been ever so gracious throughout all the stuff I had been through thus far, offered to pick up Janet and me to head over to the UCSF-Mount Zion Cancer Center for an evening cancer support session—the one that Aileen tipped me off about. To me, driving across the Bay Bridge has always been a bit of a hassle, and this was no different, with the exception that this time I was not doing the driving. Still, worse than the driving in San Francisco, where it seems that every other street is one way, is the parking dilemma. Simply put, it's horrible! As I see it, it's horrible now, and always has been! I always wondered who designs these things. Whoever it is must have one sadistic sense of humor! Anyway, we finally arrived near our destination at UCSF and pulled into a relatively nearby parking lot, where we could expect to get gouged a tidy sum parking the car for a session that's to last a couple of hours. Then, the three of us hoofed it about a block or so to where the support group session was to be held.

As one might expect, there was a large turnout for this session, headed by UCSF Clinical Psychologist Andy Kneier, and as we're waiting for things to begin I got the opportunity to visit with Aileen, who was also present.

As the session began, one by one, each person sitting in a rather large circle told their story. Each one had to decide what personal information to share. Some got very emotional; others stuck just to the facts, ma'am. At first, I felt that there was a certain awkwardness, especially to the emotions that were displayed. After all, people were struggling for the right words to say about how to cope with cancer. Others began to cry or needed reassurance. Holy Toledo! Some of these conversations seemed to be as devastating as a round of chemo. But I guess the point was that spilling one's guts is supposed to have some overall soothing effect. Still, this kind of stuff isn't for everyone, and I was not convinced that it would make me feel any better.

At times it felt uneasy and uncomfortable. Yet, in an odd way, being in the room listening to others might have actually helped me feel more secure and confident about myself. Heck, after hearing all these sob stories what could be worse? Still, I felt pretty good about myself as I decided that this really wasn't my bailiwick.

When the session was over it became obvious to me that each person experiences cancer as a unique individual, and no rigid communication rules can ever universally apply. Some people feel awkward when asked to talk about their cancer in a room filled with strangers, and though well meaning, many say things that hurt or mystify more than they comfort. At least in this environment each person could empathize with each other's circumstances. Heck, that's a far cry from trying to talk about one's cancer with another person who is totally disconnected, and responds to your comments with something well-intentioned, yet stupid, like: "Don't worry, you'll be fine."

Exhortations about being positive have their place, yet, in the end, when it comes to staying connected, it's what is in your heart that is far more important than what you say. Having friends and family that you know will be there for you and will stay the course is what really matters.

Throughout history, cancer diagnoses have often not been communicated to patients for fear of distressing them. Families have often times avoided talking about a loved one's cancer altogether. Even the word "cancer" was often unspoken, conveyed instead through euphemism or coded as "the big C." So communication and staying connected is key in helping to lift one's spirits and staying on course to help fight this dreaded disease. And that's what I aimed to do.

As the session ended and everyone dispersed, I thought to myself that this was all well and good, but I can't see schlepping myself to San Francisco for these sessions on a continuing basis. For one, the group is quite large so it lacks intimacy. Second, because of the size of the group, the time each person can speak is therefore limited. There had to be a better alternative.

So for the next few weeks I spent some time checking out other cancer support groups, including one in nearby Pleasant Hill (another generic support group that catered to the needs of cancer patients of all types but didn't have a single melanoma patient among its members) and Sacramento (just too damn far to go for a meeting and hear people spill their guts about their woeful medical conditions, and then have to drive home at night for close to two hours while in a state of depression). No thank you! What would be a better option? I'd have to give this some serious thought.

CHAPTER 5
DEALING WITH ANXIETY

The one common denominator that I observed in all the group sessions that I had been attending is that people in all of them were not afraid to express their anxiety… and boy, did they have lots of it. Not everyone, mind you, but enough to take notice. I'm certainly no expert on the subject, but that said, there are two issues that should be addressed: How to cope with the anxiety associated with having to deal with the reality of having cancer, including melanoma, and knowing that having this disease affects more than just the patient—it also consumes those close to you.

Many people easily fall into a state of anxiety just knowing that they have melanoma or perhaps another lethal disease. Heck, some have anxiety just when they take certain medical tests, like CT scans. Anxiety is very different from garden-variety nervousness. It has the power to knock some people down and keep them down.

Getting a diagnosis of metastatic melanoma, anxiety is one of those emotions that is inevitable. It's not a matter of beating or "getting rid of" anxiety. It's more about knowing that one has to learn how to live with it, preferably in peace and with acceptance.

I believe there are ways to acknowledge anxiety while not letting it take you down. Here's are some suggested coping skills:

First, don't deny it. Anxiety has a sneaky way of taking over one's mental existence, and thereby sucking the life out of you.

Some may feel that simply by acknowledging one's anxiousness by expressing yourself is a perfect outlet to restore calm from within. Yes, some may feel that expressing sadness, fear, or anger is a sign of weakness. In fact, the opposite is often true. It's much harder to express powerful emotions than it is to try to hide them. Hiding your feelings can also make it harder to find good ways to deal with them. There are many ways to express your feelings. Find one that fits you. You might try to talk with trusted friends or relatives, or keep a private journal. Some people express their feelings through music, painting, or drawing. In other words, simply acknowledging the emotion helps. It won't make it go away, but it lets you see this is not a new feeling and that you know what it is and how to handle it better.

Taking it a step further, learn as much as you can about your cancer and its treatment as possible. Some people find that learning about their cancer and its treatment gives them a sense of control over what's happening and therefore helps relieve anxiety.

Get physical. It's no big secret that exercise can make you feel better (and experts think it might also specifically help with cancer treatments), but for many it is a mental health requirement. Getting one's heart rate up for 30 minutes every day is a surefire way to control one's anxiety about treatments. Because it releases a slew of feel-good hormones, exercise helps control the negative emotions that come along with any serious health diagnosis. When I was unable to exercise for such a long period of time while being on an interferon treatment, anxiety could have easily taken over at every one of my health-related appointments. However, once I was able to begin physical exercise it made a significant difference in my outlook on life.

Choose mindfulness. There are number of meditation practices, such as yoga, that can be particularly helpful in calming oneself when the feeling of anxiety rears its ugly head. It slows the breathing, allowing for more calm.

Also, reach out to others. There may be times when finding strength is hard and things feel overwhelming. It's very challenging for any one person to handle having cancer all alone. Try to widen your circle by reaching out to friends, family, or support organizations. These people can help you feel less alone. They'll be there to share your fears, hopes, and triumphs every step of the way.

Try to focus on what you can control, not what you can't. I know that it's easier said than done but finding ways to be hopeful can improve the quality of your life, even if it won't determine whether you'll beat cancer. Despite what you may hear, people's attitudes don't cause or cure cancer. It's normal to feel sad, stressed, or uncertain, and even to grieve over how your life has changed. When this happens, expressing those feelings can help you feel more in control rather than overwhelmed by your emotions. It also frees up energy for all the other things you need to handle.

Above all, Take care of yourself. Take time to do something you enjoy every day. Cook your favorite meal, spend time with a friend or loved one, watch a movie, meditate, listen to your favorite music, or do something else you really enjoy. It will take your mind off of negative thoughts, even if it's for a short period of time. In other words, give yourself a break!

I know that living with cancer anxiety is an ongoing experience. What works for someone now may not work in six months, but with luck, one will find something that does work. In the meantime, I'll do everything I can to practice what I preach.

There's one last thing that absolutely can't be overlooked. Cancer often affects more than just the patient; it also affects family roles and routines. One's family may need to help you with or even take over things you once handled alone. You and your loved ones should talk about what changes need to be made to your family routines. This way, you can make decisions as a team and work together. Working as a team helps to make everyone more comfortable with the changes that are part of family life.

It's true that you might not be able to do all the things that you used to. You may be afraid that you'll become a burden to your loved ones, but don't think that way. Instead, talk with them about what you can do, and keep trying to do what you can. You and your family should also keep doing things you used to do together—such as playing games or just taking walks. These are healthy and fun ways to keep working as a team.

Okay, that's the lecture for the day. Now back to the subject at hand—the cancer support groups. The various support sessions I had been attending certainly had their place, but being as generic as they were, trying to appeal to cancer victims of all kinds, they were kind of like a melting pot and just didn't address the specific issues that one may hope to see should everyone in the group have a common core issue.

Hmmmmm... as Newman (from the "Seinfeld" TV show) might say, it is quite the conundrum. I was certain I could come up with something, but the timing would have to be right.

CHAPTER 6
LET'S GET PHYSICAL!

Meanwhile, we were closing in on the end of July, and upcoming was my first scheduled appointment to meet with Physical Therapist Phil Zarri. Let's face it—I was a physical mess—tilted head and all, and I needed someone to help get me get back on the right track. Phil is this really cool guy who goes out of his way to make one feel comfortable. He has the ability to tell you how messed up you are in such a diplomatic way as to actually be inspiring.

Seeing Phil was obviously a good idea. First, any exercise that he could recommend would do more than keep me fit; after all, exercise releases "endorphins," the brain chemicals that resemble morphine in their ability to lift one's mood. Also, he could certainly help to get my head screwed on straight again.

Well, I know that I looked like a long-term project. As previously mentioned, if nothing else, I hoped to just get my head screwed on properly again (literally). Hey, I had nothing but time—I was convinced of it! So Phil gave me some exercises to do. Knowing it was going to be a slow process we took it slow and easy at first so as to cause no further damage. I guess the goal was to turn my noggin into a bobblehead, if you know what I mean, so that ultimately it would turn in all directions. I was given instructions regarding exercises to do at home each day to loosen up the neck muscles and help give me more flexibility. Since I couldn't turn my neck it was impossible for me to drive. As a matter of fact, I ask you to try *not* turning your neck and see how limiting it can be on doing day-to-day things we all take for granted.

The challenge was before me—do the exercises and get this old neck working again. Does anyone have any WD-40? Nah, I guess that would be cheating. So I spent considerable time working the neck to the point that it became a rote exercise. I was acutely aware that this would be a long, arduous process; not something that would miraculously take care of itself overnight.

As time passed we entered the first of August, and it was a doubleheader day—I was scheduled to see Phil Zarri so he could check on my progress, as well as Dr. Cohen. It became evident that the program Phil prescribed aimed at me taking it slow and easy, much like the hare and the tortoise, because I was not going to get it together all that quickly. Luckily, the home exercise program he gave me used little or no equipment, so hopefully my perseverance would be the key to further the improvement of my condition. I was also encouraged to visit the Kaiser Hospital gym to use the available equipment.

Later that same day the visit with Dr. Cohen was pretty standard stuff. I was there just to get the "oil and water" checked… you know—make sure the ol' ticker was sound and that all the slicing and dicing I had experienced hadn't affected anything else. As with the rest of the physicians looking out for me, Dr. Cohen is very personable, and just like the rest of them, I believe they like seeing me because I'm always accompanied by Janet. At least that was my take on it. Hey, I don't blame them; it's just the way I saw it.

CHAPTER 7
CHOOSING A TREATMENT

On August 7 I had another scheduled follow-up appointment with Dr. Rasgon. Everything seemed to be in order, but he reminded me that the surgery was just the first step—I then had to make a decision on what treatment to choose to ensure that any possible remaining cancer didn't spread. I assured him that I hadn't forgotten, and that when I saw Dr. Simons next this subject would be of primary concern.

Another week went by and before I realized it, it was already August 15—time to see Dr. Simons for yet another follow-up. There were so many follow-up options yet so little time. All the experimental options could drive someone crazy. Who's to believe? What might really work? Let's face it, melanoma is tricky, and perhaps we are beginning to know its secrets thanks to the tireless efforts of researchers and the commitment of thousands of patients who enroll in <u>clinical trials</u>.

It's true that we are finally beginning to see true advances, but at the same time there's something baffling about this disease, and even though we are now seeing an explosion of new studies, new drugs and new promise in this field, at the time I was not completely sold. I was convinced that ultimately melanoma will become a manageable and curable disease, but at that point in time… well, I knew we were not quite there yet. To be honest, it can all be very confusing. After all, a lot of these clinical trials sounded a little like voodoo treatments.

I was aware that in rare cases where basal cell or squamous cell carcinoma has begun to spread beyond the local skin site, the primary tumors are first removed surgically. Then patients may be treated with radiation, immunotherapy in the form of <u>interferon</u>. I also knew that according to research, responses to this therapy could be short-lived. In other words, there were really no truly good answers.

So after careful thought I finally opted for the conventional protocol of one year of interferon. According to John Kirkwood, M.D., at the University of Pittsburgh Cancer Institute (UPCI), interferon extends overall survival and relapse-free survival in patients with high-risk melanoma. According to a study, high-risk patients have a 50 to 80 percent chance of disease recurrence without adjuvant treatment, or additional treatment after surgery. Furthermore, once melanoma recurs, it is often more difficult to treat. For me, having this disease once is enough. So I decided to play the odds rather than becoming a guinea pig for some completely untried and untrue other option.

During the first month of this 12-month long treatment, of which the first month involved high dose interferon, I visited Kaiser five times a week, Monday through Friday. Then, for the next eleven months, it was three days a week of low dose interferon. I knew it wasn't going to be fun, but I was determined to make the best of it. As I previously mentioned, my Grandma was a fatalist. I guess so am I. You know—what will be, will be (sort of like Doris Day used to sing: "Que Sera, Sera"). In any case, as I already said, that meant I'd be coming to Kaiser for an hour or so every single weekday, Monday through Friday, for a month. Hey, what else did I have to do, right? Okay, let's do it!

The following week—August 22 to be exact—it was time for the high-dose chemotherapy treatment to begin, and was to last every weekday for one month. So I went to Kaiser's Oncology Department where I was greeted by a couple of nurses who tried to put me at ease by explaining the routine that would be followed. I could see that there were a bunch of Lazy-Boy-style chairs lined up against the walls, and, for the most part, the patients in these chairs receiving treatment looked like ghosts from Christmases past. Well, I could see that this was going to be fun!

So the nurses found me a spot and got me started by first explaining the procedure in an effort to ease any trepidations I might have. Then they took out this gigantic needle that looked like it was meant for the giant of "Jack and the Beanstalk" fame (just kidding!) and injected me with my first dose of interferon. Basically, I just sat there for an hour while the stuff penetrated into my system. I guess the shock of this high-octane stuff was supposed to scare the melanoma out of my system. At least that's the theory as I saw it.

In actuality, the interferon treatment I had signed up for included an injection into a vein (who doesn't look forward to that?). The side effects can vary from person to person, and can include fatigue, vomiting, nausea, diarrhea, hair loss or mouth sores. Oh joy! Now these are things I could really look forward to experiencing.

At the end of the session the nurses told me 'I done good.' They would see me tomorrow for more of the same.

At first I didn't feel any after-effects of the interferon. But then it hit me. That first night was brutal—I got a fever of 103 or 104 and felt like absolute shit. It got so bad that Janet had to call the night nurse at Kaiser to figure out how to control the fever as I was sweatin' up a storm. You know what they say—"if the disease don't kill you then the cure just might!" Man, it sure felt that way that night.

Well, the advice nurse at Kaiser was extremely helpful, essentially telling me to use a cold compress and "not to sweat it." Somehow, I managed to make it through the night, wondering if this was going to be an ongoing process of 'living through hell.'

The following day I returned to my new home-away-from home—the Oncology Department at Kaiser, where I was able to meet the head pharmacist, Henry Lew, as well as Betsy, one of the senior nurses. All the folks who work in this department really go out of their way to make patients feel as comfortable as possible, and in my case, because of my ongoing number of visits (five days a week for a month) I got the opportunity to know some of them on a more friendly basis.

For some reason I couldn't get over looking at the other patients who were being treated, and noticing how gaunt they looked—almost like the walking dead. Is this the way I looked? I felt tired, but far from dead.

the process began again. This time they injected a type of drip system into my arm so they could leave it there for the entire week. If I was to take a shower my arm had to be wrapped so as not to get wet. Then I sat in one of those cozy armchairs for an hour while the chemo went through my system. Good times! To pass the time I brought a CD cassette with music that my son prepared to help me relax. I then just closed my eyes and let the hour pass. It was not too difficult a task.

As one might imagine, during that first week of the interferon treatment, I was getting phone calls from concerned friends just to find out how I was doing. It's funny, but when people called to ask how I felt, they really didn't want to hear the truth. For example, telling them: "Well, this morning I had a massive vomiting session and didn't make it to the toilet in time. Oh yeah, and I also have nosebleeds, feel bloated, and even lost a couple of pounds. I have trouble getting around because I'm so weak and have dizzy spells when I try to move too fast. Other than that, I'm just fine and dandy. And how are you?" Instead, it was just easier to tell them that I was doing okay.

CHAPTER 8
EAST BAY MELANOMA
SUPPORT GROUP

By now early September arrived and it was time for another doubleheader, including a standard follow-up with Dr. Cohen just to make sure everything was in order. Also, I saw Dr. Rasgon that same day. By now Dr. Rasgon and I could really converse in a frank manner about any range of matters. So during this visit the ol' lightbulb in my head came on. There's no rhyme nor reason for how one thinks, but for some reason I decided to mention the support group meetings I had been attending. Then it dawned on me—Dr. Rasgon was the perfect one to mention the idea of forming a fledgling new melanoma support group. It would be a local, primarily East Bay group, strictly for melanoma patients, and also very low-key in presentation and nature. I mentioned it to Dr. Rasgon, who was in a position, if he agreed, to mention it to some of his other patients, and see where it might take us. As it turned out he thought it was a good idea, and agreed to help by passing the word on to those patients of his that might benefit from such a group, and have them get in touch with me.

Later that evening I phoned my friend Aileen and mentioned my idea to her, hoping to get her input. Not only was she onboard with it, her excitement about starting an East Bay Melanoma Support Group (which is what we decided to call it) was invigorating, and all of a sudden I became more excited about it than even I thought I could be. Apparently, a few of Aileen's friends were in the same boat, recovering from melanoma, and would much appreciate having a group that could understand what one goes through in dealing with this disease. We talked about how it would be constructed, yada, yada, yada, and before too long Aileen thought it a good idea to present our thoughts about the group to some of those she knew.

So what would be our next step? Recruitment of prospective members? Okay, so how do we get them? Those were good questions. As Fagan said in the movie "Oliver": "I'm reviewing the situation. I think I'd better think this out again!"

Time had passed and it had now been about three weeks into the high dose chemotherapy routine so Henry, Betsy and I talked about continuing with the low-dose chemotherapy for the next 11 months, which was standard practice for this treatment protocol. Their preference (standard practice, whatever that means) was to have me self-inject three days a week for the next 11 months. Whoa, Nellie.... self-what??? Are you kidding? I'm thinking: "What are my other choices? How 'bout if I poke myself in the eye while I'm at it?" What other alternatives are there? Well, they tell me that I can continue coming to Kaiser three days a week and they'll "do the damage" for me.

Obviously, hauling myself to Kaiser three days a week for 11 months would seem to be a lot more inconvenient, but it was an alternative method to having to stick myself with a needle all these times. My question was what I would do on holidays and other days that the Kaiser offices are closed. After all, I was not to miss *any* days of injections.

Luckily, one of Janet's friends was a nurse, who happened to live nearby. So we asked her if she might avail herself to jab me on those occasions that Kaiser offices were closed. Not a problem—she was more than willing, and certainly able. So we settled on a long-term game plan. The folks at Kaiser would get to see my smiling face three days a week for the next 11 months—lucky them!

September 22 arrived and I was to begin 11-months of low-dose chemotherapy. To be honest, it was quite a relief to continue going to Kaiser and seeing all the staff with whom Janet and I had become well acquainted. They were all really great and eager to please. Instead of considering the trek to Kaiser a task, it became merely an hour of the day I put aside as part of my daily ritual. No big deal! I would go in, exchange pleasantries, get my injection, and say *'sayonara!'* until the next day's treatment.

One of the pleasant side results of this otherwise tedious, yet necessary experience of being a constant visitor to the Kaiser Oncology Department was the opportunity to get to know some of the staff. I've previously mentioned Henry, the department's chief pharmacist, who is a cool guy—one with whom you can easily have conversations, whether it be pharmaceutical matters, sports cars (he loves Porsches) or just every day life. Another, whom I've also mentioned, is Betsy, a department nurse, who is both caring and cheerful. They, along with many of the other department nurses, made coming each day much more than just tolerable. They were able to put each of their patients at ease, despite going through this grueling treatment. Strangely enough, going each day was something I could actually look forward to doing—not because of the injections (I'm not a complete idiot), but rather, because of the welcoming personalities.

By the beginning of October I was scheduled to see Dr. Mark Reisman, Head of Dermatology, for a full body check. It might have seemed a little like letting the horse out of the barn after it's already burned to the ground, but it really wasn't. Dr. Reisman is very thorough, and at the same time very approachable. I would point to things that by now might seem like a bit of paranoia, but he would spend the time to explain exactly what each mole was. Basically, I didn't have any moles that were worth worrying about, but at the same time, I knew I had to remain vigilant not to let any new moles go unnoticed or ignored. I did not want to go through what my dad did, having a dermatologist that told him about questionable marks on his skin by saying to him: "If it doesn't bother you it doesn't bother me." Yeah, we know how that turned out. So instead of scheduling annual visits, I was to come in to be reexamined every few months—just to be on the safe side.

Because I was still under tight scrutiny, I got to visit Kaiser twice more this month; on October 6 to see Dr. Rasgon (I was confident that him seeing Janet's smiling face just made his day!), and two weeks later to see Dr. Cohen. Seeing this team of doctors had become a routine part of my existence. Still, quite frankly, because each of them was so concerned about my recovery, yet at the same time low-key, they had gained my complete trust.

By early November I was scheduled for a Dr. Simons follow-up appointment. As with Dr. Rasgon, Dr. Simons and I were on quite friendly terms and could talk openly about a lot of stuff. So I decided to mention the idea of our new, fledgling melanoma support group and asked if he could mention it to any of his patients in oncology that might want to inquire more about it. As with Dr. Rasgon, he was onboard.

Slowly but surely both Aileen and I began to get phone calls inquiring about the support group. I found it amazing how much each person had to say about their individual circumstances and how eager they were to share details. It became clear that just the emotional well-being of having the opportunity to spill one's guts about such traumatic circumstances of having melanoma could be so cathartic. It became evident that the beauty of such a support group would be that each person could speak openly or ask questions about what was going on and the others could all directly relate.

Interestingly, it's my opinion that the timing of starting the East Bay Melanoma Support Group was fortunate since there were so many clinical treatment choices. Decisions! Decisions! I hate to put it this way, but one person's positive potion may be another person's poison. Even the so-called experts couldn't be sure what was best on a person-to-person basis. Anyway, having others' support and the opportunity to voice one's concerns was a step in the right direction.

By now it was back to physical therapy, and because of what Aileen and I were establishing, I felt pretty upbeat. Phil Zarri could see that I was making progress. I realized that getting everything back in order would not happen overnight, but I had lots of patience. After all, I didn't plan on going anywhere soon, if you know what I mean. Phil saw my exuberance so he allowed me to go to the Kaiser gym whenever I wanted and he told me what exercises would be best. *All right*—progress was being made—small steps, but nonetheless, I was heading in the right direction!

CHAPTER 9
SEEING THE 'JOLLYTOLOGIST'

On November 15 I decided to go visit with the Kaiser Cancer Support Class, and much to my pleasure the topic was uplifting. The guest speaker was Allen Klein, whose official title is "Jollytologist," and has won awards for his "Going After Laughter" presentations. The room was packed, which told me (as if I didn't already know) that people with diseases would really rather hear a speaker with a positive, even light-hearted message, than one who is both matter-of-fact and perhaps even depressing.

In any case, there were lessons to be learned from Jollytologist Klein, and while he had the audience cracking up with his antics, I took some life-lesson notes. His basic topic was "Humor: How to Use It to Get Healthy and Stay Healthy." Sounds good to me!

This guy (pardon the pun) was "just what the doctor ordered!" He reminded us that while the world is usually viewed as a serious place, filled with job hassles, family strife, traffic jams and other 'stressors' that threaten our mental and physical health; often the best defense is also the most fun—a good sense of humor!

There's no doubt that humor gives you a new perspective on life. It reduces psychological stress and makes it easier to cope with difficult situations. And it can break the cycle of negative thoughts one tends to dwell upon, as well as anger and anxiety.

Laughter also has physiological benefits. Did you know that blood pressure and heart rate rise briefly during a hearty laugh, then drop below their original levels? That's the same thing that happens during aerobic exercising. In fact, one humor researcher calls laughter "internal jogging." Laughter also helps loosen tight, tense muscles.

Recent research suggests that laughing also boosts the immune system. What's the evidence? Well, supposedly, blood levels of the stress hormone 'cortisol' drop when one laughs, while levels of 'T cells' (natural killer cells), antibodies and other immune system components increase.

Humor is especially important for people facing serious illnesses. Let's face it; a good laugh is a welcome distraction from the pain and strain of a serious illness.

You've probably heard the story of Norman Cousins, the magazine editor who aided his recovery from a life-threatening illness called 'anklosing spondylitis' by watching videotapes of the Marx Brothers and the Three Stooges. Hey, I'm not saying humor is a cure-all, but, as my father-in-law would say, "It can't hoit!"

Interestingly, in recognition of the healing power of humor, many hospitals now offer humor rooms and humor carts with funny books, comedy tapes and humorous videos. A few even have closed-circuit comedy channels.

So the prescription offered at this session was evident: Don't take yourself too seriously, and be sure to incorporate humor into your daily life. After all, it's impossible to overdose on laughter. It gives you a certain degree of power over your specific situation.

As I like to say about humor therapy: it's no joke! Cancer humor therapy involves using humor, laughter, jokes, and all-around funny stuff to help relieve stress and pain. It's an actual complementary cancer therapy that's often used in addition to cancer treatment and can be as simple as watching a sitcom or a favorite screwball comedy. The goals of cancer humor therapy are to boost mood, encourage relaxation, reduce stress, and generally improve one's quality of life.

Although humor therapy doesn't improve cancer outcomes, it can help you better cope with pain, give you an improved sense of well-being, and provide a welcome respite from the seriousness of cancer and its treatments.

One study did find that laughter can actually improve immune function, which is important for cancer patients battling the disease and trying to heal their bodies during cancer treatment.

Stress is a definite detriment to physical and mental health, and lots of laughter is a great way to combat it.

Oh, and I might add this small tidbit: When choosing a doctor, make a real effort to find one with a good sense of

humor. You'll feel more relaxed and closer to a doctor who not only understands you but is able to share laughs with you. You'll relate to each other as real people and find it easier to work together to find that path to real health.

CHAPTER 10
MY HOME AWAY FROM HOME

From that day forward I became a regular at Kaiser, whether it was to see one of my doctors or to attend one of the cancer support group sessions. Between that time and the end of my chemo sessions in August, 2001 I saw one doctor or another for a grand total of close to 30 times—that included getting update checkups about three times per month—and that didn't include the trips to UCSF to see Dr. Mohammed Kashani for even more checkups! Either they really didn't believe I was going to make it or they thought I just might be a freak of nature! I'm really not sure which it was. Regardless, I felt pretty fortunate that I was still here and kickin'!

Summer ended with little fanfare, and the Fall season was actually very pleasant; no medical setbacks of which to speak. Then, early during the Thanksgiving week it was time to attend one of the Cancer Ed Support Group meetings—I had just attended another Kaiser Cancer Ed Support Group session, but my mind wandered (nothing new about that—just ask my wife!). I kept thinking how differently I would propose having the meetings of the East Bay Melanoma Support Group since most of the people in attendance at these meetings were just sitting around. After all, these sessions were open to people with any form of cancer and therefore the content of discussion was often generic.

Within days the phone started ringing much more than expected (many phone calls had been directed to Aileen), and by now we actually believed we had enough people to schedule the first meeting of the new East Bay Melanoma Support Group! It would be an informal setting, with dinner included, and everyone could mingle and introduce themselves, telling their personal story in as much (or little) depth as they chose.

As time evolved the group continued to grow, personal friendships were cultivated, and the topics and depth of scope were astonishing. Various members were trying so many different treatment options. What it told me was that *no one*—not even the so-called experts—had a handle on what was the best method to attack melanoma. It was strictly a crap-shoot. Even another doctor, one from Children's Hospital, joined the group, and was able to give others in the group a different perspective—one from a doctor who is now an 'insider.'

While we were all at risk for melanoma at varying degrees, it was clear that some were more at risk than others. One topic that our group raised was that of heredity. If one's mother, father, siblings, or children have had a melanoma, you may be part of a melanoma-prone family. Further, if melanoma occurred in a grandmother, grandfather, aunt, uncle, niece, or nephew (second-degree relatives), there is still an increase in risk, compared to the general population, though, granted, it is not as great.

About one of every ten patients diagnosed with melanoma has a family member with a history of the disease. If melanoma is present in one's family, you can help to protect yourself and others by being particularly vigilant in watching for the early warning-signs, when it is easiest to detect.

So, Thanksgiving was upon us and after a wonderful day of *gobble! gobble!* in which the family got together in a Norman Rockwell fashion, it was then time to get back to reality. That means a post-Thanksgiving visit to see Dr. Rasgon, followed the very next day with a Cancer Ed Support Group session. Again, Dr. Rasgon was pleased with my progress as there were no noticeable signs of anything spreading or of anything new appearing.

The topic at the Cancer Ed Support Group session, as with all the previous sessions, was pretty generic. Just as all cancers are not alike, treatments and side effects for various types and stages of cancer are different. They talked about treatments, which can involve chemotherapy, radiation therapy, surgery, alternative medical treatment, and other methods. As one may expect, side effects, too, can be different. It was good to hear about these things, but I preferred to hone in on the specifics of melanoma by hearing from others who are experiencing similar issues.

Time began marching on more quickly than one can imagine, and before you knew it winter was in the air. At the year-end East Bay Melanoma Support Group session one of the topics we discussed was skin care. I can't stress this enough—because I hate stressing— the sun is not always our friend! Yes, it is a great source of vitamin D. But there is a deeper, darker side that cannot be overlooked. Not only can it kill you if you are unprotected, but it causes wrinkles— and who wants to look like a shriveled-up old grape? Protecting your skin needs to be at the top of your to-do list when outside. Melanoma is one of the most common cancers in women under 40 and is responsible for 80 percent of skin cancer deaths. So pay attention! Use sunscreen! How long before you reapply the sunscreen? Often! I'd say about every hour and a half. Applying it more frequently dramatically reduces your burn risk. The problem is that most of us in the East Bay Melanoma Support group weren't diligent about applying sunscreen growing up, and the results had taken a toll. So whether you're hitting the beach, lounging around or spending the day outside, remember to layer on the lotion. And for those of you still trying to catch rays indoors, stop! People who use indoor tanning machines have up to a 75 percent increased risk of melanoma. In fact, some of you ladies might even recall using cocoa butter to "cook," I mean tan, properly. Well, that's a no-no!

So the week before Christmas I paid a holiday visit to see Dr. Cohen. Although he's not in his Santa suit he still came across as jolly. As always, he was very welcoming. Again, I'm pretty sure it's because Janet was with me. In any case, he checked the "oil and water," if you know what I mean, and I somehow passed inspection. It was a very good way to end the year.

The holidays that year were pretty uneventful—just the way I like it, and before I knew it we were in a new year! Of course that meant that I was back getting checked out at Dr. Rasgon's office on January 3, 2001. Well, happy New Year to me!

This was just the first of a barrage of appointments I had as the New Year began. I was getting checked out just about on a weekly basis from an entire team of skilled and concerned Kaiser physicians. First up was a melonama checkup with my dermatologist, the incomparable Dr. Reisman. Did I mention what an unheralded behind-the-scenes "star" this guy is? Apparently, back in the day he had a school friend who eventually became a writer for the "Seinfeld" television series.

Well, the two of them stayed in touch through the years and when they got together for lunch one day they talked about dermatology. Apparently his friend was so intrigued by what Dr. Reisman was saying that it became the groundwork for what was eventually to become "The Slicer" episode for the "Seinfeld" television show in which Jerry and Dr. Sara Sideridis (Marcia Cross) are having lunch (just as Dr. Reisman was with his friend) when a former patient thanks Dr. Sara for saving his life after battling skin cancer. Dr. Sara says, "Do you have any idea what it feels like to save someone's life?" Jerry responds, "Is it anything like hitting a homer in softball?" Later that day when Jerry is chatting with his friend George Costanza about his time at lunch he says: "Saving lives? She's one step above working at the clinique counter. Dermatologists? Skin doesn't need a doctor." George responds, "Of course not. Wash it, dry it, move on." Later in the episode when Jerry visits Dr. Sara in her office he confronts her by saying: "You call yourself a life saver? I call you Pimple-Popper, M.D." Check it out for yourself.

CHAPTER 11
NO NEWS IS GOOD NEWS

The following week it was back to see Dr. Cohen for yet another checkup. I wasn't exactly certain what they were looking for since everything seemed to be in order, but I guessed it was better to be safe than sorry. In any case, I passed the test... this time.

Before you could blink an eye February arrived and I had so many doctor appointments scheduled that they were coming out of the ol' wazoo. On February 7 I saw Dr. Rasgon; followed two days later with an appointment to see my oncologist, Dr. Simons. Then the following week I had a follow-up MRI on the slate. That's always a fun time. They stick a needle in your arm for contrast, and then slide you inside a skinny tube. It's a good thing that I'm not claustrophobic.

As if that wasn't enough, five days later I got a CT Scan, to be absolutely certain that I was not going to the dark side. Then, on February 26 it was time to see Dr. Rasgon again to review all the test results. Things must have been looking pretty good as there was no cause to change any of my protocol. The following day I saw Dr. Cohen again and got a double stamp-of-approval that things were going in the right direction. While I still lacked any real stamina or energy, I knew that slow and steady was the right course of action.

As the first week of March approached I was back in Dr. Rasgon's office. I'm guessing that he took great delight in squeezing my neck, looking for anything suspicious, just to watch me cringe. It was literally a pain in the neck when he felt for any lumps or irregularities. Luckily, he found none.

That same week the East Bay Melanoma Support Group convened once again. One of the topics discussed was that of CT scans. Doctors today are using CT scans more than ever. If used at the right time and for the right patient, they can be lifesaving. On the other hand, it seems that doctors are ordering those radiation-emitting tests more often than might be required, exposing patients to high rates of radiation; clearly a health danger. Most patients substantially underestimate the level of exposure they receive, and most believe that they are unaware of any risk of it actually causing cancer.

Radiation from CT scans—each of which is equivalent to 100 to 500 chest X-rays, might contribute to thousands of estimated future cancers a year. Yet some hospital systems and some doctors continue to order them more often than necessary, exposing patients to needless risk and expense.

At the group meeting we discussed how many health care providers have little knowledge about radiation and thus are poorly equipped educators. Obviously, it's a doctor's job to ensure that patients are aware of the benefits and risks of their recommendations. Some of the group's conclusions included: a) If one's doctor orders a CT scan, ask whether magnetic resonance imaging (an MRI) or an ultrasound can be done just as effectively instead; b) Be wary of double scans. A double CT scan, one with a contrast agent and another without, can offer useful information, but it's not usually needed, nor worth the risk; c) When in doubt always get a second opinion.

April 5 comes and it is a splendid occasion as it's a "twofer"— that's right, I got to see both Dr. Reisman and Dr. Rasgon. Oh joy! I got the privilege of being probed all over two times that day! Fortunately, as they say, no news is good news.

During the months of May and June I got the privilege of seeing Dr. Rasgon, Dr. Cohen, Dr. Reisman, and Dr. Rasgon once again, all as part of a continuing effort to be vigilant in making certain that there were no new developments.

Then summer finally arrived and the East Bay Melanoma Support Group met once again. Being diagnosed with melanoma can be disorienting, frustrating and often bewildering. For most people, when first told that "you have melanoma" it is something one never dreams they would hear from their doctor.

Sadly, studies show more and more people are being diagnosed with this disease. In fact, one in 50 Americans may be diagnosed with the potentially deadly cancer in their lifetime. The increase in these numbers shows three things:

First, we need new and better treatment options for people diagnosed with melanoma. Second, we must expand our efforts to prevent the disease in the first place. And finally, people affected by melanoma need greater support systems to accommodate the increasing need for information and comfort.

From a preventative standpoint, one can certainly be more vigilant about checking themselves. After all, when a melanoma is detected at an early stage, a cure is is much more favorable. The key here is that one must know what to look for. There are some basic warning signs, which have conveniently been named the "ABCDs" so that they can be easily remembered:

"A" stands for Asymmetry. Basically this means that if you could draw a line through the middle of the melanoma, the two sides would not match. This is in contrast to a benign mole, which is round and symmetrical.

"B" stands for Border. Melanomas are usually irregular in shape, often times with ragged edges. In contrast, a benign mole has smooth, even borders.

"C" stands for Color. Melanomas show a variety of shades of brown or black; sometimes even with shades of red or even blue. They are really ugly. By contrast, common moles generally have a uniform brown color to them.

Finally, "D" stands for Diameter. A melanoma is usually at least the size of a pencil eraser. While there may be exceptions, if you find that you have a mole this size or larger be sure to have it checked out immediately. There's no sense taking any chances.

The long and short of it is that self-examination can save your life. The old saying goes, "If you can spot it, you can stop it!" In other words, performing self-examination of one's own skin, like when you take a shower, is highly recommended, especially for those who are at risk of getting melanoma, whether by genetics or otherwise.

In my case, spotting the melanoma was quite difficult as it was located at the crown of my head, completely covered by hair. Hey, at least I had my hair! In any case, when showering I felt an odd shape at the crown and this is when I decided to visit Dr. Liss in the first place. Lucky I did.

One really doesn't need any elaborate equipment to conduct a self-examination. Having a full-length mirror is always good. A hand mirror can give you a close up of any moles that you wish to examine more closely. If that isn't sufficient, you can always ask your spouse/significant other to examine you. Granted, I admit that it's not very sexy, but it can be life-saving.

Then, at each subsequent self-exam be sure to look for any changes in size, shape or color. Some new moles may even have appeared since your last self-exam. Be sure to take note of those little buggers. You could even take a photo and email them to your dermatologist for review, thereby saving you yet another expense and trip to the doctor's office.

One of the most important things is not to jump to any conclusions after conducting a self-exam. It reminds me of that old Arnold Schwartznegger movie when he says, "It's a too-ma!" In other words, because you may see a change in one of your moles, do not immediately jump to conclusions that you have a melanoma. Some moles may look dangerous, but in reality they are benign. On the other hand, some look benign, but may be more dangerous. Confusing enough? Only a physician can tell one from the other for sure, so if you see a suspicious-looking mole, get it checked out by a professional.

In any case, by now it's June 27 and I got a good report after seeing Dr. Cohen. He's my internist; not my head and neck guy, mind you. But still, I was getting a little bit of my energy back and I was beginning to feel pretty good.

Putting things in perspective, it was clearly a shock to first learn of my diagnosis of having melanoma as I did last year. Obviously, there was a lot of worry and life-altering decision-making that had to be made. It all makes one have a certain amount of introspection. So I made a list of little things that can be reminders that you are a cancer survivor or heading in that direction:

1. Your alarm clock goes off at 6 a.m. and you're glad to hear it.
2. You're back in the family rotation to take out the garbage.
3. You no longer have an urge to choke someone who says, "all you need to beat cancer is a better attitude."
4. Your dental floss runs out and you buy 1000 yards.
5. When you use your toothbrush to brush your teeth and not comb your hair.
6. You have a chance to buy additional life insurance but you buy a new car instead.
7. Your doctor tells you to lose weight and do something about your cholesterol and you actually listen.
8. Your biggest annual celebration is again your birthday, and not the day you were diagnosed.
9. You use your Visa card more than your hospital parking pass.

CHAPTER 12
AN EYE TO THE FUTURE

Realizing how short and precious life truly is, and fully realizing that there is a "dark period" one must maneuver through, I along with Janet, made a decision that if and when I got healthier and garnered a bit more energy, there was no reason to keep our dreams on hold. So we decided it was time to have a change of scenery and do some leisurely travelling.

We both like cruising, and it is easier on the body to travel in this fashion, having others wait on you, than say, to go camping or do something strenuous in the rugged outdoors. No thank you to that. I prefer: "Oh Jeeves! Oh Jeeves! Another Perrier, if you don't mind." Yes, that sounded a lot better than sitting in a tent on some windy mountaintop looking over your shoulder to see if there are any bears or other varmints nearby.

So it's decided that we would head to New York to take a cruise up the eastern shore, all the way to Montreal. There are a number of ports that we had never visited before, and it would be fun. More important, it would be a celebration of lasting through a year of dealing with a dreaded disease and finishing what seemed like a treatment marathon that in and by itself had taken its toll, both physically and emotionally.

Dealing with future issues and events are commonly put off indefinitely. In this respect my struggles may have actually been a blessing. Clearly, dealing with things for the present, rather than the future, would not have occurred had I not had to face a potentially life-threatening disease, and for that, I am thankful!

As the month of July approached we celebrated Independence

Day in a most traditional way—by attending a local town parade, followed by a barbecue. As always, and most important, it was a time to spend with family. What can be better than that—presuming everyone gets along?

In keeping with the Red, White and Blue theme, when the East Bay Melanoma Support Group convened during this month an obvious topic was one that is all too frequently ignored—skin care. Here are some basic tips that members of the group chimed in as key to help prevent skin cancer:

1. Always apply sunscreen: Sunscreen is something that needs to be applied year-round, and yes that means even in the winter! You can wear a moisturizer that contains SPF protection and make sure to apply your sunscreen 30 minutes before going out in the sun and then again every 2 hours after that. Don't forget to apply it to your ears!
2. Wear clothing with UPF protection: You can protect your skin by keeping covered and wearing special clothing. When you're out in the sun, SwimZip is a great choice of UPF 50+ swimsuits, swimwear, and accessories for kids and adults.
3. Keep your head covered: Wearing a hat will cover areas that are hard to apply sunscreen to, like your scalp, ears, and neck. It will also protect your face more than just with sunscreen alone.
4. Take a break from the sun when out: Never stay out in the sun all day long. You should seek shade during the afternoon when the sun's rays are at their strongest.
5. Check for signs: Check your skin and be familiar with your moles so if you see anything new or changing you can see your doctor and detect skin cancer at an early stage when it is most treatable.
6. Be consistent: Make applying sunscreen part of your daily routine with your kids so they can pick up the good habit. They will know to never leave the house without applying sunscreen and it's also a time to educate them on skin cancer awareness.

By mid-month it was time to see Dr. Simons again. Since the oncology department was already my home away from home this was hardly a big deal. Besides, he seemed always grateful when I showed up for my appointments—and had Janet accompany me! He wanted to know how I was handling the interferon and if there were any lasting side effects. Aside from not having any stamina or energy, was boredom a side effect? Other than that, the plan was to stay the course.

A week later I saw Dr. Rasgon, who checked everything out to make sure that everything was in place. This guy knows so much, but what is so great is that he has the ability to articulate things in a manner that his laymen patients can understand. So he explained a little bit about skin care by the numbers. Interesting stuff. It's always good to know some basic stuff:

* The number 2—That's the number of spots you need to double-check on your self-skin exam. For girls, it's the calves. For guys, it's the back. But really, it's important to check everywhere, even areas that have never been exposed to the sun like the bottoms of your feet or in between your toes.
* The number 50—That's the SPF value you should be wearing everyday and everywhere, especially during summer months. SPF 50+ is the gold standard when in the sun for a prolonged time. What it really comes down to is the label, in addition to 50+, you want to see claims like "broad-spectrum sunscreen offering protection against both UVA and UVB rays." UVB rays, the ones SPF addresses, are responsible for burning skin, but UVA rays penetrate deeper into the skin and cause aging.
* The number 85—That's the number of minutes you can spend in the sun before reapplying sunscreen. The reasoning here is simple. Melanoma often arises in areas that have had sunburns and especially among people who have had numerous sunburns. Applying your sun care more frequently dramatically reduces your burn risk.
* Finally, the number 800—This is the percentage that Melanoma has increased in young women over 40 years. Yes, natural skin is the new tan. So whether you're hitting the beach, lounging poolside, or simply spending the day outside, remember to layer on the lotion.

And for those of you still trying to catch rays indoors, stop! People who use indoor tanning devices have up to a 75% increased risk of melanoma.

On August 8 I was then scheduled to see Dr. C. J. Morton for a follow-up PT Scan. Just to be clear, a PET scan (PET stands for positron emission tomography) uses radiation, or nuclear medicine imaging, to produce 3-dimensional, color images of the functional processes within the human body. Basically what happens is that the machine detects pairs of gamma rays that are emitted indirectly by a tracer, which is placed in the body on a biologically active molecule. The purpose is to find out how an existing condition is developing or how effective an ongoing treatment is working. In my case, despite a lack of energy (which my wife constantly tells me I have anyway, especially when it comes to doing chores around the house!), I felt like I was on the right course—at least I hoped I was.

So after the prepping, I was taken to the room where the PET scan is taken, and told to lie down on a cushioned examination table. The machine had a large hole, kind of like a tunnel, which the table slides into. If you are claustrophobic then you would not appreciate this exam. Luckily, I just closed my eyes and pretended that I was somewhere—*anywhere*—else. Then the images of the body were taken and before you knew it, it was all over.

I had wondered what the differences were between a PET, CT and MRI scan, especially since I had to utilize each of them during my ordeal. Basically, a CT or MRI can assess the size and shape of body organs and tissue. However, they cannot access function. A PET scan looks at function. In other words, MRI or CT scans tell you what an organ looks like, while a PET scan can tell you how it is working.

My doctors had covered all the bases, giving me each of these exams, and therefore, they knew the makeup of my body—ounce by ounce.

A few days later the East Bay Melanoma Support Group convened once again, and a primary topic is once one gets this dreaded disease, how does one develop a positive outlook? This can be quite the conundrum since having melanoma can suck the life out of you—if you let it!

For some, being hopeful once one learns that he has melanoma, is not easy. Still, many melanoma patients succeed in developing an optimistic outlook. I feel one almost has to do it in terms of becoming self-rewarding in terms of happiness and mental outlook (which is also good for your physical, not to mention one's emotional health). From a clinical perspective, those who reject depression, despair and self-defeatism have a better chance of survival. You've got to want to kick melanoma right in the rump, having no second thoughts about it.

Still, having a positive attitude to conquering this disease is certainly easier said than done. So what can one do to get onboard with this strategy? First, accept your doubts and fears as the normal reaction to learning that you've got cancer. You needn't keep these feelings to yourself. Hey, that's exactly why the East Bay Melanoma Support Group came into existence.

Belonging to a group, or even talking to a friend, neighbor or relative who understands your situation and concerns is a true comfort, especially to those who are anxious (and who can blame them?). Welcome whatever support they may offer.

Having an understanding spouse is invaluable (thank you Janet!). Marriages and any of these other relationships are frequently strengthened when people face this type of illness together. It's called teamwork. And it really does work.

On the other hand, for those who live alone, as millions of Americans do, today's technologies allow other forms of communication to touch base with those who might be able to understand you, no matter how far away they may be—even across the globe.

Still, having the ability to cope with anxiety associated with having to deal with this disease can take its toll, as members of our support group can attest.

Many people easily fall into a state of anxiety just knowing that they have melanoma or perhaps another lethal disease. Heck, some have anxiety just when they take certain medical tests, like CT scans.

Anxiety is very different from garden-variety nervousness. It has the power to knock some people down and keep them down.

After getting a diagnosis of metastatic melanoma, anxiety is one of those emotions that is inevitable. It's not a matter of beating or "getting rid of" anxiety. It's more about knowing that one has to learn how to live with it, preferably in peace and with acceptance.

I believe there are ways to acknowledge anxiety while not letting it take you down. Here are some suggested coping skills:

First, don't deny it. Anxiety has a sneaky way of taking over one's mental existence, and thereby sucking the life out of you.

Some may feel that simply by acknowledging one's anxiousness by expressing yourself is a perfect outlet to restore calm from within. Yes, some may feel that expressing sadness, fear, or anger is a sign of weakness. In fact, the opposite is often true. It's much harder to express powerful emotions than it is to try to hide them. Hiding your feelings can also make it harder to find positive ways to deal with them. There are many ways to express your feelings. Find one that fits you. You might try to talk with trusted friends or relatives, or keep a private journal. Some people express their feelings through music, painting, or drawing. In other words, simply acknowledging the emotion helps. It won't make it go away, but it lets you see this is not a new feeling and that you know what it is and how to handle it better.

Taking it a step further, learn as much as you can about your cancer and its treatment as possible. Some people find that learning about their cancer and its treatment gives them a sense of control over what's happening and therefore helps relieve anxiety.

Get physical. It's no big secret that exercise can make you feel better (and experts think it might also specifically help with cancer treatments and even lessen side effects), but for many it is a mental health requirement. Getting one's heart rate up for 30 minutes every day is a surefire way to control one's anxiety. Since exercise releases a slew of feel-good hormones, it helps control the negative emotions that come along with any serious health diagnosis. When I was unable to exercise for such a long period of time while being on an interferon treatment, anxiety could have easily taken over at every one of my health-related appointments. However, once I was able to begin physical exercise, it made a significant difference in my outlook on life.

Choose mindfulness. There are number of practices, such as yoga and meditation, that can be particularly helpful in calming oneself when the feeling of anxiety rears its ugly head. It slows the breathing, allowing for more calm.

Also, reach out to others. There may be times when finding strength is hard and things feel overwhelming. It's very challenging for any one person to handle having cancer all alone. Try to widen your circle by reaching out to friends, family, or support organizations. These people can help you feel less alone. They'll be there to share your fears, hopes, and triumphs every step of the way.

Try to focus on what you can control, not what you can't. I know that it's easier said than done, but finding ways to be hopeful can improve the quality of your life, even of it won't determine whether you'll beat cancer. Despite what you may hear, people's attitudes don't cause or cure cancer. It's normal to feel sad, stressed, or uncertain, and even to grieve over how your life has changed. When this happens, expressing those feelings can help you feel more in control rather than overwhelmed by your emotions. It also frees up energy for all the other things you need to handle.

Above all, take care of yourself. Take time to do something you enjoy every day. Cook your favorite meal, spend time with a friend or loved one, watch a movie, meditate, listen to your favorite music, or do *anything* you really enjoy.

I know that living with cancer anxiety is an ongoing experience. What works for someone now may not work in six months but, with luck, one will find something that does work. In the meantime, I'll do everything I can to practice what I preach.

There's one last thing that absolutely can't be overlooked. Cancer often affects more than just the patient; it also affects family roles and routines. One's family may need to help you with or even take over things you once handled alone. You and your loved ones should talk about what changes need to be made to your family routines. This way, you can make decisions as a team and work together.

Working as a team helps to make everyone more comfortable with the changes that are part of one's family life.

It's true that you might not be able to participate in all the things that you used to. You may be afraid that you'll become a burden to your loved ones, but don't think that way. Instead, talk with them about what you can do, and keep trying to do what you can. You and your family should also keep doing things you used to do together— such as playing games or just taking walks. These are healthy and fun ways to keep working as a team.

From my own experience, I found that members of the East Bay Melanoma Support Group recognized the importance of attempting to confront one's anxious behavior, no matter how difficult it may be. It's certainly a step in the right direction.

During the month of August and early September I had follow-up appointments to see Dr. Cohen, Dr. Rasgon and Dr. Reisman. Well, the bottom line could be simply stated by that old standby once again—"no news is good news." At least that's the way I interpreted the results of these visits. Looking back, while one can never be too careful, as I've learned during this journey, I remained hopeful. So instead of dwelling on what "might be" I continued to take a more positive approach and focus on where I stood at this point in time. After all, it had been over a year since the original diagnosis, and I was still around and kicking in spite of the odds against my being here.

CHAPTER 13
TIME TO CELEBRATE!

September 9 arrived—Admission Day—so Janet and I celebrated the anniversary of the state of California joining the union as we began our journey by leaving the Golden State to go to New York. Oh yes, not to be forgotten was that it was also a celebration to mark the occasion of my beating the odds by surviving cancer for one year. Hey, it's a start, and one really doesn't need a reason to celebrate anything. But if there's anything worth celebrating, it's the idea of kicking cancer in the pants—even if it's only been for a year. I couldn't get it out of my head that I was given a 7 percent survival prognosis, and yet here I am!

So we headed to New York, which was where we were to board a cruise ship that would take us through New England and conclude in Montreal. We knew it would be a grand time.

We spent a day sightseeing throughout New York before we boarded our ship at the New York port. Later that evening, around 10 p.m., I decided to take one final view of the city from the deck level. I had my movie camera with me, and got some great panoramic shots. As it turned out, they are memorable. After all, it was September 10, 2001. I may very well have been one of very last people to catch the Twin Towers on film… just a few hours later and they would be no more!

Then, the unforgettable attack on the United States on 9/11 put a deep-seeded damper on all that was to follow for the duration of the trip. Everyone on board was glued to all news updates, and the shore excursions and all that was supposed to be joyful about taking such a vacation all of a sudden took a backseat to the unfolding events of the day that shocked the world. It all really makes one pause to think about the world we live in. And I guess that's the point. The events of 9/11 were a real eye-opener. After all, life is unpredictable. One simply doesn't know what is to come around the corner, so one needs to live for today and make the most of it.

As for those diagnosed with cancer, everything changes about your life. Yes, there are those who might have a simple diagnosis, breeze through treatment and then actually get back to a normal life. But for a majority of us, the first time we hear the words "It's cancer!" is a game changer that impacts every aspect of our lives—including who we are and who we will become.

Without question there has been an unsurpassed amount of advancement in melanoma treatment research. As time marches on the progress and breakthroughs in research advancement have been unprecedented. The Melanoma Research Foundation's (MRF) funded projects have been able to address critical areas in melanoma research such as how to overcome resistance to therapies for cutaneous and ocular melanoma, discovery of new melanoma targets and drugs, a better understanding of why melanoma metastasizes (spreads), dissecting the genomic drivers of ocular melanoma, and new ways to monitor melanoma therapy.

One thing remains perfectly clear—medical progress is definitely moving forward at a rapid pace, especially in the areas of immunotherapy and precision medicine. Just a few years ago the thought that we could successfully treat half of all people with advanced melanoma would have been inconceivable. Now that such a goal is within sight, we must not forget that this amazing result still leaves many, many people struggling for better solutions. But, heck, I'm so excited about the progress and the possibilities for the future that I believe I'll hang around for a while longer just to see how things turn out.

EPILOGUE

Time has passed since I completed my treatment for melanoma. Actually, it's been well over a decade. The East Bay Melanoma Support Group that was formed years ago no longer meets. Sadly, most of its members are no longer with us. I am one of the lucky ones to still be around. As for me, well, T.S. Eliot said it best: "Every moment is a fresh beginning." Even today when I see my doctors they still have an incredulous look of amazement when I walk in the door. Why are they so amazed, I wonder? After all, it's in great part because of their handiwork that I'm still kickin'. Most of the doctors I used to see on a regular basis have since retired; while others are going as strong as ever.

Some things regarding skin cancer have really changed over the years—and for the better. Today, there is much more general awareness of the effects of being in the sun, and protecting oneself with sunscreen, etc. Tanning salons? They may still exist but the image they once had of delivering a bronzed "hip" look is long gone—a thing of the past now that people are better educated as to the harm of the rays! Today it's even recommended that little babies wear hats and sunglasses as protection from the sun. After all, one thing we have learned is that sun rays beating down on you is cumulative. The most dire effects of a sunburn come in the years before the age of 20.

In Australia, which has the dubious distinction of having the highest rate of melanoma worldwide, there is a campaign called the "3 S's" (Slip-Slop-Slap) to help protect them from rays beating down from the sun. The "3 S's" campaign, launched in 1981, even features a singing, dancing Sid Seagull, encouraging people to reduce sun exposure and protect themselves against an increased risk of skin cancer. Sid has Australians slipping on long-sleeved clothing, slopping on sunscreen and slapping on a hat. The thought of a child possibly getting skin cancer is taken so seriously that putting on sunscreen is required of school children before they are allowed play outside.

A depleting ozone layer? The general public was largely ignorant of scientific things such as this back when I was growing up. Today, there has been significant research in determining how important it is to protect oneself from exposure to the sun for great lengths of time.

Today, continuing research is still the key to understanding the mechanisms behind the disease's development and growth, and is necessary to advance the treatment of—and potential cure for—melanoma.

In 2016 alone, for example, an estimated 144,000 people were diagnosed with melanoma in the U.S., resulting in nearly 10,000 deaths. Ten new therapeutic regimens were approved from 2011 to 2015 giving hope to patients and families. Despite the advances in these new treatments, much remains unknown including how to sequence and/or combine available treatments, what allows some tumors to build up resistance to therapy, and which drugs are likely to work best with each patient.

Yes, a lot has been accomplished as far as scientific research and new treatment options since my initial cancer diagnosis, and today there are many. For years at my checkups we would ask, "are there any new treatments?" and the answer we would get was always, "not really." However, today in the fast-moving world of melanoma treatment, new options for patients with this metastatic disease are emerging faster than ever before. Still, the question exists: which should be the first line choice in metastatic melanoma—targeted drugs or immunotherapy. Eventually we will find the answer.

As for me, well, even at my now-advanced age I still get out there and stay active in part by tossing the ball around in a senior softball league. The only difference (aside from perhaps slightly declining ability) is that I'm much more aware of "preventative maintenance" when it comes to tackling melanoma. For one thing, I lather on the sunscreen before playing. Also, instead of wearing a baseball cap, now I wear one of those safari caps with a protective "drape" attached to the backside, protecting my neck. Some of those that I play with used to kid me, even in a mocking fashion by calling me "Lawrence of Arabia" because of the cap I wear that might look like I'm more ready for the Sahara Desert than to actually take the field. But even that ridicule has died down in recent times. Apparently they're catching on that protecting one's neck may not be the ultimate fashion statement, but it's the smart thing to do to avoid a melanoma diagnosis. Now I keep protected whenever I go outside. Hey, maybe I'm not so dumb after all! And you shouldn't be either. After all, as Friedrich Nietzhe once said, "That which doesn't kill us makes us stronger." Amen to that.

ABOUT THE AUTHOR

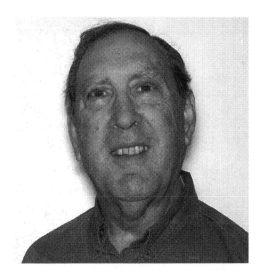

George Epstein is a native Californian and third generation melanoma victim. He organized and played in softball tournaments for decades, and remains an avid player in the senior softball circuit in the East Bay. After his diagnosis of metastatic melanoma in 2000, he continues to be diligent about covering up with his "special hat" with earflaps whenever he is outdoors. Despite the odds against him, George's unwavering optimism is an inspiration to all who meet him.

73206747R00046

Made in the USA
Columbia, SC
07 September 2019